RICHARD HITTLEMAN'S GUIDE FOR THE SEEKER

Richard Hittleman's Workshops on Monterey Bay, California, are attended by students from throughout the world seeking his unique guidance in Yoga meditation, philosophy and physical exercises. The vital Workshop instruction to which the reader might otherwise never have access is made available in this book.

Here are the fascinating teacher-student dialogues—the answers to those perplexing questions that are in the minds of all "seekers." Mr. Hittleman also presents for the first time in any book a section depicting the "correct" and "incorrect" positions of Hatha Yoga Postures.

Richard Hittleman's books, classes and TV programs have enriched the lives of millions of Americans. This book—the essence of all his teachings on Yoga—can do the same for you.

RICHARD HITTLEMAN'S GUIDE FOR THE SEEKER

Richard Hittleman

BANTAM BOOKS · TORONTO · NEW YORK · LONDON

RICHARD HITTLEMAN'S GUIDE FOR THE SEEKER
A Bantam Book/May 1978

All rights reserved.
Copyright © 1978 by Richard Hittleman
This book may not be reproduced in whole or in part, by
mimeograph or any other means, without permission.
For information address: Bantam Books, Inc.

ISBN 0-553-11171-X

Published simultaneously in the United States and Canada

Bantam Books are published by Bantam Books, Inc. Its trade
mark, consisting of the words "Bantam Books" and the por-
trayal of a bantam, is registered in the United States Patent
Office and in other countries. Marca Registrada. Bantam
Books, Inc., 666 Fifth Avenue, New York, New York 10019.

PRINTED IN THE UNITED STATES OF AMERICA

0 9 8 7 6 5 4 3 2 1

CONTENTS

Foreword

What we are searching for, we already have!

My association with Richard Hittleman has extended over a period of two decades. It has been my privilege to arrange for the publication of his books, to produce the "Yoga For Health" television series, and to assist in the scheduling of his classes and lecture tours.

In recent years, I have arranged for Mr. Hittleman to conduct a series of workshops and seminars at Pajaro Dunes on Monterey Bay, California. Students have come from many parts of the world to participate in these six-day programs, which consist of intensive training in Hatha Yoga, seminars for Yoga instructors, lectures and discussions of the principles of Yoga and Vedanta, private consultations with Mr. Hittleman, and training in meditation.

During the course of these workshops, it became apparent to me that those questions which were being asked by attending students regarding all aspects of their spiritual studies and practices, were so consistently similar that they undoubtedly echoed the questions of "seekers" throughout the world who are involved in the spiritual quest— regardless of what form this quest takes. And whereas the students in attendance were receiving direct answers from Mr. Hittleman that proved to be of great assistance to them, it may very well be that others who are involved in the quest are not as fortunate in finding satisfactory instruction.

Therefore, with the objective of making Mr. Hittleman's seminar teachings available to all who seek the illumination such teachings have provided, I recorded the six meetings of the Discussion Group at the most recent workshop. In addition to a transcript of these recordings, this book is comprised of: the procedure utilized by Mr. Hittleman in the meditation sessions; a section of photographs depicting the corrections made by instructors in the Hatha Yoga classes (which should be extremely helpful to those who are practicing the *asanas* without access to a competent instructor); a bibliography that was distributed at the workshop. Mr. Hittleman assisted in the selection and editing of all materials that appear in this book.

A few words describing the physical setting of the meetings, and backgrounds of the students, should be of interest. Pajaro Dunes is situated on the beach of Monterey Bay and is surrounded by hills and open fields. The Discussion Group met for approximately ninety minutes each afternoon. Depending upon the weather, the group convened either on the lawn or in a comfortable meeting room. Students ranged in age from twelve to eighty-two; they came from all sections of the United States and many foreign countries, and they represented numerous sects and religions. Some were absolute beginners in the spiritual quest, while others had been involved in various metaphysical and spiritual pursuits for more than twenty years; between these extremes were students in all stages of development. Dozens of occupations and professions were represented. In the overall view, the worldly lives of the students and their stated objectives in attending the workshop were so diversified (this diversity is reflected by the questions that appear in the text) that the only common denominator that could be discerned was their aspiration to be instructed by Mr. Hittleman. (It was most fascinating to observe how, during the relatively brief six-day program, the superficial objectives of certain students were significantly revised, as these students were exposed to the philosophy and techniques of Yoga.)

To make the dialogues easy to read, minor editing of the recordings was necessary: questions that were awkwardly phrased have been improved and generally clarified; questions and discussions that were irrelevant have been deleted; unnecessarily lengthy questions have been reduced to the basic points. It is essential for the reader to understand that the students asking the questions are at *different levels of development*. This variance accounts for the fact that certain of Mr. Hittleman's responses are more simple and basic than others. It also explains why some questions that are almost identical—but were asked by different students—receive different treatment.

The dialogue form—particularly that which includes question and answer—has been a revered method of instruction in the East since time immemorial. Many of the most important teachings in the *shastras* (scriptures) are conveyed in this form; the *Bhagavad-Gita* is one such work. Through the years I have observed the effectiveness of the dialogue format in Mr. Hittleman's classes: I know, without doubt, that the lives of innumerable people have changed radically as a consequence of the very type of conversations that appear in this book.

What we are searching for, we already have! is the underlying theme of Mr. Hittleman's instruction. Most of his responses to students are variations on this theme. In the following pages I have endeavored to accurately transcribe his teachings at the workshop, and I trust that the profound benefits experienced by those who attended will be shared by the reader.

—Mort Levitt
Carmel, California

RICHARD HITTLEMAN'S GUIDE FOR THE SEEKER

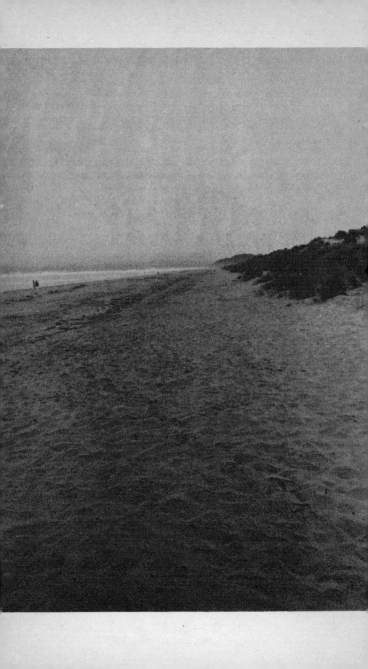

1st day

Student: I have been very unhappy for the past few years. I have read that Yoga, which leads to Self-realization, can help me change my life, so I have come here to learn about it.

RH: There is nothing to be learned about Self. Self [*atma*] is your true and eternal nature. You are now and have always been Self and you can never be anything but Self. Therefore, there is no possibility of "real-izing," that is, of making the Self "real."

Student: If I am Self then why am I unhappy?

RH: Because you have forgotten your true nature and you now believe that you are a body and a mind. Body and mind are subject to endless change. That which changes gives rise to pleasure and pain, happiness and despair. Before your present unhappiness you were happy and eventually your present unhappiness will pass, only to be followed by more unhappiness at a later time. This cycle has no end. What is constantly changing cannot be *real*. Only that which is permanent and eternal is real. Therefore, reestablish yourself in Self. This is Yoga.

Student: Does this result in permanent happiness?

RH: Yes, but not as you are conceiving happiness at this moment. The happiness, the bliss of Self, is not the opposite of unhappiness as you are presently experiencing it. Self-bliss [*ananda*] transcends duality. In your present state you know of happiness only in relation to your degree of unhappiness, and vice versa. When one resides wholly in Self, opposites do not arise; Bliss alone obtains.

Student: How could I have forgotten Self if that is my true nature?

RH: When the mind is turned outward and becomes lost in the world, Self is forgotten. The mind flows outward because one believes that his or her fulfillment lies in the world and therefore constantly seeks it there. But the wise person knows better. He or she turns the mind *inward*, finds Self, and remains there.

Another Student: If we cannot find fulfillment in the world, why does it exist?

RH: Who says it "exists"? Does the world come to you and say, "I exist"? No. You see the world so *you* say it "exists." But *how* do you see it? Are you seeing something that is really external and apart from you, or is the world that you see actually a projection of your mind, which then becomes lost in its own projection? Merge your mind with Self and then you will know if the world exists. The nature of the world cannot be Known until mind is turned inward and merges with self.

Another Student: You said that we *believe* we are a body. Do you mean that I am *not* a body? That it is not real?

RH: Let us be clear on the meaning of *real* as it pertains to our Yogic study. What is born and dies and is subject to continual change between birth and death is transient and hence unreal. Inherent in all that is unreal is pain, misery, despair, and suffering. This unreality of that which is transient is contrasted in our teaching with that which is eternal, never-changing, without qualities, and beyond duality. This eternal principle is designated "Self" and "Reality." I should point out here that we will be using the pairs of opposites such as Self and not-Self, wise and ignorant, real and unreal, only as conveniences for discussion. In the ultimate sense, merged in Self, no distinction as to what is real or unreal can arise.

The body, a temporary sheath in which you appear to find yourself, cannot be considered *real* in the sense of *eternal*. Since your true nature is that of eternal Self, you are not the body. The fact that your senses, nervous system, brain, etcetera, perform their various functions and interpret to you the experiences of an organism—pain, hunger, satisfaction, and so forth—does not mean that your Reality is that of the body. Anyone who has meditated seriously knows that he loses the sense of body during meditation. When, eventually, the body dies, the Self certainly does not die.

The ignorant man identifies with and limits himself to a body, making it the focal point of existence. He maneuvers this illusory body through an illusory world, seeking happiness, fulfillment, and peace. But his quest has no possibility of success. He is like a thirsty man on the desert who, each time he sees a mirage of water, believes it will quench his thirst. He reaches out to drink and the water vanishes. That is why the wise men speak of life that is lived in this type of quest—identifying with the body and seeking fulfillment in what appears to be an external world—as filled with incessant suffering, disappointment, restlessness, and frustration.

Student: If I am not in the body, then where am I?

RH: Yes, that is the fundamental question. Find out *where* you are.

Student: How can I find out?

RH: There are a number of effective techniques. They are all based upon the principle of dissolving the ego, which is also the mind. The mind, the thinking machine, the computer which I designate "ordinary mind" to distinguish it from Universal Mind—the unadulterated Intelligence of Self—is in constant turbulence. This turbulence is called "thinking" and is extolled by ordinary men. Quieting the mind, withdrawing it from the world (the mirage) which it projects, and tracing it to its source is what must be done.

Another Student: If we stop thinking we won't be able to function.

RH: Do you make this observation from your experience?

(The student did not reply.)

RH: You believe that you are your mind; so of course you believe that if your mind is inactivated you will also become inactive. But are you actually your mind?

Student: I've never really thought about it.

RH: Yes, that has been the case until now. But now you desire to Know Self, so now you must investigate. What you call "functioning" transpires very well, indeed, it usually transpires much better, when your identification with your mind ceases. You must recognize that you are not your mind any more than you are your body.

Another Student: You said there are a number of techniques to dissolve the ego. Which is the best?

RH: It is a matter of which is best for *you*. People are at different levels of understanding and, therefore, require different techniques.

Student: How will I know which is best for me?

RH: Do you meditate?

Student: Yes, I've been doing it for about four months. I repeat the *mantra* "I Am That." I do this for about thirty minutes in the morning and again in the evening. [*Editor's note: a* mantra *is a formula composed of a special arrangement of syllables and is used for purposes of incantation.*]

RH: Are you dissatisfied with this *mantra*?

Student: It helps to quiet me but I can't judge if I'm progressing.

RH: Well, of course you must understand what is to be accomplished by your repetition [*japa*] of the *mantra*. The *mantra*, as with other techniques, gives the mind something upon which to fix so that other thoughts are excluded. If thoughts arise, the mind dismisses them as quickly as possible and returns to the *mantra*.

Through this process, the mind gradually becomes steady and one-pointed. Nothing can be accomplished until the mind is brought to this one-pointed state. However, when this state *is* attained, the student must understand that it is not the ultimate objective. Now the consciousness must merge with Self. In your case, your *mantra* must lead you to the recognition that you are *not* "that." You are not "this" or "that" or *anything whatsoever!* The Truth is that you simply ARE. Therefore, the *mantra* "I Am That" must evolve into the recognition of "I AM."

Student: And this recognition occurs naturally?

RH: Yes, but by "naturally" we do not mean that it happens without effort.

Student: Do you recommend that I continue with this *mantra*?

RH: Where did you get it?

Student: It was suggested by a former teacher.

RH: Can you now, at this moment, apprehend your true nature? Can you recognize *who* you are and *where* you are?

Student: (After a pause): I don't feel it.

RH: Then continue with your *mantra* . . .but with your full attention and awareness. Do not allow the repetition [*japa*] to proceed automatically like a child who recites a portion of the Constitution without knowing what he is saying.

Student: Couldn't I now drop the "That" and just use the phrase "I AM"?

RH: You stated that your *mantra* had been given to you by a teacher and I have no wish to disrupt whatever relationship you may have with him or her.

Student: There was no real relationship. It was just her suggestion. I don't even know where she is now.

RH: Then you may utilize "I AM." You may find it more effective without the objectification of "That."

Another Student: About what you just said a moment ago: If I can grasp *who* I am and *where* I am, can I give up meditation and all other practices?

RH: If you knew who and where you were, this question would not arise.

Student: You are primarily an instructor of Yoga. It must be your conviction that Yoga is the best path.

RH: Yoga encompasses many avenues and many techniques. There are the physiological and esoteric paths of Hatha and Kundalini Yoga; Jnana Yoga, which is the path of knowledge; Bhakti Yoga, the path of love and surrender to God; Karma, the Yoga of action without attachment; Raja Yoga, which is the synthesis of these and which carries the seeker to the ultimate state. Therefore, in my view, there is no path that cannot be considered Yogic.

Yoga is the mergence of what, at this moment, you think of as "I" with Self. Yoga is both the means and the goal of this mergence. When it is said that a person is "practicing Yoga," what is meant is that he or she is using the *techniques* of Yoga to *achieve* Yoga.

In Reality, however, there is no mergence. There is only Self. Because in one's ignorance [*avidya*] one has the illusion that he or she is separate from Self, we speak of "mergence." In Self there is no possiblity of the existence of a separate "I". Only Self EXISTS; only Self IS. When one recognizes Self, one sees no other. What you now conceive of as the world, is Self. All creatures, people, things, and conditions in all the universes are only Self.

Another Student: Does one retain any sense of individuality in the mergence?

RH: Why do you ask?

Student: I'm attempting to visualize what this ultimate state is like. I'm trying to feel what it would be like if I lost myself.

RH: There is no possibility of "loss". Loss and gain are fantasies of the ordinary mind. But all such speculations as to what the enlightened state [*samadhi*] is like are meaningless and consume time that could be devoted to practice. Consider the peculiarity of what you just said: "I am trying to feel . . .something, something . . .if I lost myself." How many *I*'s do you count in this statement? There is the I who is "trying to feel" another I who may lose its "self." So there are two *I*'s and a self. Where did you get all these personal entities? Which of these is your *real* I? your *real* self? Investigate. You can make this question, "Which is the *real* I?" the seed of your meditation. This questioning, seriously pursued, will reveal the illusory nature of what you cherish as "I."

Another Student: Although you said that you viewed all paths as "Yogic," there are many other paths with different names that are followed by people who may never have even heard the word "Yoga." Is the goal the same in all these manifold paths, systems, and methods?

RH: Yes. The means may be multiple, but the goal is the

same for all. There is only one ultimate goal: recognition of Self.

Another Student: Here, at the workshop, we have Hatha Yoga classes three times each day. If the body is illusory, why do we devote all this attention to it?

RH: Hatha Yoga is a remarkable path to mergence with Self through the body—not the gross body, but the subtle body. As the classes proceed, you will be instructed in the pertinent details. All the physical exercises [*asanas*] and breathing techniques [*pranayama*] are practiced toward that end. The physical health and well-being that are experienced through this practice are by-products. The Hatha Yoga system is primarily concerned with the transcendence of the "I."

The Hatha practice strengthens and purifies the *subtle* body through the techniques performed by the gross (physical) body. The objective of this process is to enable the subtle element *prana* to be directed into a channel [*nadi*] where it ordinarily will not go. The entrance of the prana into this channel has a two-fold effect: first, the thoughts cease and the mind is at rest; second, a unique energy [*shakti*] which lies dormant in a sleeping but potentially active state is aroused. This is the energy or shakti which is designated *kundalini*. When activated, the kundalini is led by the student through a series of centers [*chakras*] and made to unite with the energy of Siva. This unification is actually the mergence of the "I" energy [the kundalini] with the energy of Self [Siva]. Thus, Yoga is achieved: the I is dissolved in the Self-experience.

Student: Then what becomes of the body? Does the "I" consciousness return eventually?

RH: These discussion sessions are not a suitable format in which to present the technical details involved. Students in the intermediate and advanced classes will be instructed in these matters. Others can read of the system in my *8 Steps* book. [*Editor's note: see the bibliography.*] The point I wish to make here is that Hatha

Yoga should be understood as a system that directs the student to the experience of Self. The physical benefits are by-products.

Another Student: I've always thought of Hatha Yoga and Kundalini Yoga as two separate systems.

RH: Technically, this separation may be made. Today there are numerous teachers throughout the world who are instructing Hatha Yoga without knowledge of its ultimate objectives. They do not know about the application of *kumbhaka* [breath retention], *mudras* [gestures], and so forth, for the purposes of arousing kundalini. Certain teachers attempt to arouse kundalini without the preparation of Hatha. But the great ancient gurus of Hatha make it very clear that the objective of Hatha is to arouse kundalini so that Self is experienced. Those of you who are interested in learning of the ancient teaching along these lines can study the source works: *The Hatha Yoga Pradipika, The Gheranda Samhita*, and *The Siva Samhita*. [*Editor's note: see the bibliography*]. However, those who are not attracted to the Kundalini practice may, nonetheless, utilize the Hatha techniques to prepare the consciousness for other avenues of meditation.

Another Student: Is it all right to change paths, that is, to try different methods?

RH: If you are attracted to a particular path you must test your fitness and aptitude for it by devoting yourself seriously for a reasonable period. In this way, you will determine if it is the path for you to pursue. Otherwise, you will run from one system to another, from one teacher to another, from one retreat to another, and you will derive little. This is exactly what is happening to many thousands of seekers, especially those who are young.

Student: Last year you stated that Hatha Yoga can be practiced by *all* seekers regardless of what other paths they are following.

RH: In my experience, Hatha—even in a modified

form—has proven a pleasant and productive method for a great many people. The major elements of Hatha are the body and the breath. Frequently, the elements involved in other systems are more abstract and elusive, and therefore are not easily grasped. But the body and the breath are known to all and that is why Hatha can provide an excellent introduction to Self-knowledge. Everyone can move the body and, to some extent, control or at least *observe* the breath. These things are of great assistance in learning how to make the mind one-pointed.

Another Student: I've found that about fifteen minutes of Hatha Yoga and then a few minutes of Alternate Nostril Breathing greatly improve my ability to meditate.

RH: Yes, there is no doubt of that. The *asanas* remove tension that is associated with stiffness and promote the free flow of energies. So the body becomes less of an encumbrance. Then, Alternate Nostril Breathing, or just the simple observation of breathing, quiets the mind and prepares it for the one-pointed state that is a prerequisite for meaningful meditation. It is in this sense that Hatha can be an important adjunct to all other paths.

Another Student: When I lived in New York I was a student of Zen for a short time. My *roshi* [teacher] described Zen as being different from any other practice.

RH: In techniques, yes; in objective, no. Self is the goal of all.

Student: One of the students there became my good friend. She had been practicing for nine years and she told me that she had not reached *satori* [*samadhi*, Self].

RH: No matter how many years a person practices, she will never *reach* Self. If we had to *reach* Self this would imply that Self is somehow apart from us, that there are two selves—one that has to reach the other. Are you two selves? Of course not. Self is not something to be arrived at, or something to be acquired. Self is your original, true, and only condition. We practice not to *reach* Self but to remove those fantasies and illusions that obscure it.

Student: Perhaps I misquoted her. I'm not really sure she used the word *reach*, but my point was that nine years seems like a long time. Shouldn't she have achieved the goal?

RH: We cannot conjecture about such things. The element of time does not enter into the meditation practice. We do not attempt to meet a deadline in Yoga, Zen, or related practices. We practice without the anticipation of results. What we think of as "progress" in the world does not manifest in the same way in the meditation practice. And nine minutes, nine years, or ninety years is of no consequence. The business of your life is to recognize Self. When this is achieved, you understand that you have always been Self and whatever "time" has been spent in this achievement has no meaning. Indeed, time itself will be recognized as an illusion.

Student: So she could be approaching the goal and not know it?

RH: There is no point to such speculation. . . . Were you involved in Soto or Rinzai Zen?

Student: Rinzai.

RH: Her *koan* has been given to her so that she may come to understand the illusion of the subject-object relationship. That is, I (subject) do not *see* the flower (object). I AM the flower. The flower and I are Self. One may comprehend this intellectually, but one must come to Know it with one's complete being. Only her roshi can evaluate what "progress" she is making toward this end. The roshi will guide her. [*Editor's note: the Zen koan is a question or problem given to the student by the roshi and becomes the seed for the student's meditation.*]

Another Student: Is breath control used in Zen?

RH: Becoming aware of one's breathing by fixing the attention on it is a practice of many systems of meditation. But, whereas in these systems only the simple *observation* of breathing is suggested, in Hatha Yoga the regulation and control of the breath has become an entire science. This science is known as *pranayama* and is comprised of a series of breath-control techniques.

Another Student: I frequently hear and read that "time is an illusion" and you said the same thing a few moments ago. I cannot really understand how time can be an "illusion." You can't deny that there are past, present, and future, and that anything that "happens," that is, any event, takes place in time. It is now three-thirty in the afternoon and the sun will be setting at about five-thirty. Is this an illusion? Tomorrow morning we will be attending the Yoga classes at seven-thirty. Is tomorrow morning an illusion?

RH: "Time" is one of many elements that have been devised by ordinary mind as an expedient for coping with situations and conditions in the world it projects. Time is a tool of ordinary mind and can be utilized as such. But *you* are not transient. You are Self. Self is eternal and cannot exist in time. When you manifest Self, it appears to the ordinary man that your body acts and moves as if it were adhering to the time element, but in Reality time no longer exists for you.

You exist only as Self, and Self exists only NOW. NOW does not mean the "present" in terms of the past-present-future sequence. Now is NOW. NOW IS ALL. NOW IS SELF.

Another Student: You know, as you were just speaking, I grasped the truth of what you are telling us, and it really is strong. It pushes me out of my self. I had this feeling when I read the same information that you gave about "time" in one of your books. But just a few moments later I lose it and I'm back in time.

RH: Ask yourself, "*Who* is back in time?" A transient "I" can appear to move in time, but how can eternal, unchanging Self exist in time? Are you not eternal Self?

You cannot be "in" time and then "out of" time. Find out *who* is having the dream of a time dimension.

Another Student: The science-fiction authors write about weird things that happen when people get into different time dimensions.

RH: All "time" is the same regardless of the dimension. The most incredible science-fiction story of all is the illusion perpetrated by your ordinary mind. It conspires to have you think of yourself as that which you are *not*; and that which you *are*, it prevents you from knowing. What could be more "weird," more totally "fictional," than that?

Another Student: We're always thinking about the past, aren't we?

RH: Note what you have said. You said "thinking" about the past, not *experiencing* it. You can think about the past, but you can do that thinking only NOW. Do you ever remember a time that was other than NOW? You can also "think" about a "future," but you can only do such thinking NOW. The future never comes. And if you lend credence to the past-present-future sequence, how can you exist in the present when the present has already lapsed into the past? No, you EXIST only NOW as SELF.

Student: Why don't I really *know* that?

RH: Find out *who* it is that says she doesn't know.

Student: What is your opinion of TM [Transcendental Meditation]?

RH: My "opinion" is of no consequence. It is what it is. If a system is comprised of the pure teachings, it will prevail. I define the "pure" doctrine as one that propels the aspirant relentlessly and unswervingly to the recognition of Self. If the doctrine is not of this nature, then millions of dollars spent on promotion and publicity cannot secure its survival. Countless such systems and organizations have come and gone. Do not concern yourself with these matters. Attend to your own enlightenment.

Another Student: Is it necessary that a mantra be given by the guru, or can a person just choose a mantra that attracts him from a book and meditate with it?

RH: If a seeker is seriously attracted to a system in which mantra is the major element—that is, if he is serious about pursuing the path in its entirety and is not simply playing with the mantra because it is currently the "in" thing to do—then the mantra must be transmitted by the guru. The dynamics of mantra are extremely subtle. Mantras are like magnets which draw the student to Self. Classically, a relationship is established between the aspirant and the guru and the guru ascertains the aspirant's level of understanding before the appropriate mantra is transmitted. The guru invests the mantra with power and this power acts as a catalyst to activate the mantra. Only a true guru, one who has himself attained enlightenment, has the necessary authority and power. Without this authority, the mantra may be effective in quieting the mind and senses and imparting temporary tranquility, but it cannot provide the ultimate experience, which is to pull the student into the mantra to the extent that he *becomes* the mantra and remains in the *samadhi* state [Self]. At all times, the guru is sensitive to the aspirant's development and provides the necessary guidance [*upadesa*]. The guru continues to "push" the seeker from without, while the mantra "pulls" or "draws" him from within.

Student: Where does one find genuinely enlightened gurus of mantra?

RH: If it is necessary that you find such a one, he will appear.

Another Student: How can you judge if a person who is giving the mantra is really qualified? I mean, he can say that he is and that he belongs to such-and-such an organization and has been trained by such-and-such a teacher who is the disciple of a person who is the disciple of a guru, but how do you actually know?

RH: Trust your intuition. Your intuition is the real guru within who always guides.

Student: I must tell you that I am now using a mantra, but I do not feel that the person who gave me the mantra has the qualifications you outlined. Should I continue with the mantra?

RH: Question the one who has given you the mantra.

Student: What if his answer doesn't satisfy me?

RH: Once you have chosen a guru, you must trust him or her implicitly. Whatever response is forthcoming to a question must be accepted. If you do not have such trust, then this is not the right guru for you.

Student: What if the person who has given you the mantra tells you that he has the authority to do so but that he does not claim to be a guru in the classical sense?

RH: Then, as I have said, the mantra can produce only partial results. Also, you must understand that the repetition of a mantra for a few minutes a day, without undertaking the accompanying aspects of mantra—a way of life—is a dubious and fragmented effort. This is like a man taking several headache tablets each morning and evening to relieve the pain, but neglecting to determine the *cause* of his headaches. In this way, the mantra becomes a palliative, not a cure. If the mantra is being utilized in the "palliative" manner, you can arbitrarily apply the word *transcendental*, but in Reality the mantra cannot act to "transcend" ordinary mind in the permanent, ultimate sense.

Another Student: I don't fully understand why the mantra would be less effective when given by one person rather than another. The syllables and the sound are the same regardless of who gives them.

RH: Well, there are several essential things to be understood here. First, a mantra is not simply an arrangement of syllables; it is a source of energy which will not fulfill its ultimate purpose unless it is properly activated. Second, the guru cannot be considered an ordinary man or woman. To the eye of one who does not recognize the guru's attainment, he may appear to live and act as an ordinary man; but, having transcended body, mind, and ego, the guru is no longer subject to those laws which govern the man who is ignorant of his true nature. As such, the guru has both the authority and the power to guide those seekers who are in search of Self.

I'll give you an example of what I mean by "authority." Let us say that you walk into a police station. You point to the sergeant sitting at the desk and you issue this command to a nearby policeman: "Arrest that man." The policeman looks at you in astonishment and you repeat the command: "Arrest that man." The policeman, of course, takes no action. But the sergant becomes concerned as to your sanity and, fearing that you are up to no good, points to you and issues this command to the policeman: "Arrest that man." At once the policeman takes you into custody and shortly thereafter you find yourself behind bars. The command that was issued by both you and the sergeant was identical. But only the sergeant had the *authority* to precipitate the action. In this same way does the authority to activate the mantra rest with the guru.

Another Student: In your books* you suggest that the student use the mantra "OM." Doesn't this also require a guru?

RH: OM is an all-inclusive mantra. OM is everything. It designates the creation, preservation, and dissolution of the universe. As such, it can be utilized to advantage as the seed of one's meditation. It can be undertaken without direct transmission from the guru. However, you must remember that the repetition of OM does not

---

Guide to Yoga Meditation and *Yoga: The 8 Steps to Health and Peace.*

imply that you are involved in the total system of Mantra Yoga, which requires that one adhere to the total Patanjali structure. This is an appropriate time to tell you that Ramana Maharshi considered "I AM" [AHAM] to be the supreme mantra. It is the name of Self or God, and one who intones this mantra is proclaiming that Self is his true nature. "I AM" is Self-evident.

Another Student: I think it might have been Krishnamurti who said that if you repeated the phrase "Coca-Cola" it would have the same effect as a mantra.
(Laughter)

RH: Yes, the same effect as a mantra not transmitted by a guru. If you wish to determine the effect that a mantra produces, you may experiment with OM, or with I AM, or you can sit quietly for several minutes each day and simply repeat your own full name. . . . I see some of you are smiling, but be aware that your name *is* a mantra permeated with the essence of your being, and it can be extremely effective in quieting the mind and imparting an interval of tranquility. Always remember, however, that quieting the mind and lowering the rate of the pulse or heartbeat is a temporary expedient. The thoughts will soon arise again, the illusory world will seem real and command your attention, and Self will not be recognized. *Relaxation is not Recognition.*

Student: Can you explain further why you say that fulfillment is not possible in the world? I believe I have known quite a few periods of fulfillment in my life.

RH: The fulfillment, peace, and happiness that you say you have known and that everyone knows at one time or another are transient. Your fulfillment is incomplete because however fulfilled you think you are, you soon find yourself needing additional fulfillment. Whatever peace of mind is experienced soon degenerates into new turmoil; one's peace cannot become permanent in the world. That is why you say that you have "known quite a few periods." If you had truly Known Fulfillment, you could not speak in terms of the recurrence of fulfillment.

Happiness is sought by everyone, and people engage in every imaginable activity in order to experience what they conceive constitutes happiness. But, because *change* is the nature of the ordinary mind, the world which ordinary mind projects is an entity in which all things are forever changing. Therefore, happiness which is gained through activity or acquisition cannot long remain. Those conditions and qualities which now make something attractive and desirable, something worth the devotion of all your attention, are changing; since the conditions and qualities are impermanent, the attraction cannot endure. Therefore, the ordinary man's *new* attractions—the desire for new possessions, new situations, new activities—are endless. Consequently, he suffers interminably, because each time he believes he is on the verge of finding happiness, or that he has actually grasped it, it either dissolves altogether or moves, tantalizingly, just out of reach. As often as this occurs, he *still* believes that he can capture whatever it is he is seeking. He is very slow to realize that his situation is like that of a man attempting to pick up a handful of water. He does not recognize that ordinary mind, the entity that is sending him on the endless wild-goose chase after happiness in the world, is the same entity that is projecting the world! The Reality is that Bliss is man's true nature; he need not look for this Bliss in an external illusion, but need only manifest as Self.

Student: Then why can't we just do it?

RH: Not *do* it. There is nothing to do. BE IT.

Student: It's difficult.

RH: It is not difficult and it is not easy. It just IS. What can you ever be, other than Self? Find out *who* is saying "it's difficult."

Another Student: But being happy and sad, and experiencing suffering and peace, is life. That's what life is.

RH: Nonsense. That's the bill of goods you've been sold.

Does life come to you and say, "My nature is to be happy and sad, and you are to direct your activities in experiencing my happiness and sadness?" No, *you* have decided that such is the case, or rather it has been decided for you.

Student: By whom?

RH: By the collective ordinary mind of man, of which your own is a part. All those who are ignorant of Self, their true nature, live in the condition of *maya*. Maya is a Sanskrit word that designates the state of existence in which a man forgetting his true nature, Self, identifies himself with a mind that is attached to a body that exists in a world. He permits this "mind" to maneuver this body through this world in a quest for happiness, fulfillment, and peace. The quest is futile because the realm in which it appears to be taking place is unreal, as we have already discussed. This unreality or illusion is what is denoted by the word *maya*.

Student: Is it the mind that's the culprit?

RH: The mind, the thinking machine, the computer which I refer to as "ordinary mind" to distinguish it from Pure Intelligence, appropriates unlimited power and, falsely acting as an omnipotent guide, convinces you that if you will follow its directions it will lead you to fulfillment. Because you have been conditioned since the time of your birth and in countless previous lifetimes to believe that happiness, success, and fulfillment are the true goals of life, you permit yourself to fall under the spell of the ordinary mind and be hypnotized by its endless promises. The fact that you, and all with whom you come in contact, never achieve that happiness which has been promised does not deter you from continuing the endless activities that are dictated by ordinary mind. When, time and time again, you fail to achieve the ultimate peace, happiness, and fulfillment that are promised, you are convinced by ordinary mind that your failure is due to circumstances, bad luck, destiny, incompetency, karma, and so forth. You fail to place the blame where it lies: you do not recognize that *what the ordinary mind has promised, it cannot deliver*! It is an entity that computes, that has the capacity to deal only in statistics and qualities, regardless of how profound, complicated, or abstract these statistics and qualities may be. As such, it is absolutely incapable of providing the fulfillment it promises. Its ingenious treachery lies in the fact that it is able to convince you again and again that it *can* provide what you seek. Early in life you are taught to depend on this ordinary mind to make all things possible and to place your unqualified trust in it. Indeed, you worship it. "The mind of man!" you exclaim. "What is beyond its ability?" Your trust in it is continually reinforced by all people with whom you come in contact. Everyone is seeking happiness and everyone is relying upon his ordinary mind to furnish the necessary directions. So, of course, you go along unquestioningly.

Student: Sure. You can't even begin to believe that everyone is wrong.

RH: It's not as much a question of "wrong" as it is an unintentional conspiracy or "put-on." Each man puts the next man "on" through a sort of "Emperor's New Clothes" syndrome. Each man speaks to the next in terms of the various ways in which to find happiness and satisfaction in the world. No one says, "Hey, wait just a moment. What if all these things we're doing and acquiring and thinking don't lead to what we *really* want and *really* need? What if our *minds* have been misleading us all this time?"

Student: That's a difficult conclusion to arrive at. If you can't trust your mind, who can you trust?
(Laughter)

Another Student: Suppose you *do* reach that conclusion—then what?

RH: Then you have "awakened" from the dream; the illusion begins to dissolve; the snake begins to turn back into the rope. You become a seeker. You may be led to Yoga or a related practice. If so, you will be instructed in those techniques which investigate the nature of ordinary mind.

Student: Then what becomes of the mind? Is it no longer functional?

RH: It has never been functional. To understand this you must know what the mind *is;* you must find out from where it arises; you must perceive its nature.

Student: But if you investigate the mind, don't you use the mind itself for the investigation?

RH: Yes. The nature of the mind is known through its investigation of itself! To accomplish this, the mind must turn *inward*. When the student persists in this inward turning of mind to investigate its own source and nature, it is illuminated by Self.

Another Student: You said before, "Know what the mind is." Who does the "knowing?" Does the mind "know" itself?

RH: Let us put a capital *K* on that word and say "Know." The ordinary mind never Knows anything. It can only know *about* things. It can never wholly and completely apprehend something and Know its nature, because it can never *merge* with anything. Its function is to analyze, distinguish, examine, differentiate, investigate, judge, and so forth. To function in this manner necessitates a subject-object relationship with everything. That is, no matter how subtle or abstract the examination, it must remain outside or apart from that which it examines. But, in order to grasp the essence of anything, it is necessary to merge or accomplish Yoga with it. The mind and senses can inform you of the shape, odor, color, texture, and taste of an apple. But these are only qualities, things *about* the apple. What is the *essence*, the principle of the apple? To know this, one must *become* the apple. In becoming the apple, the subject-object condition is dissolved. Since the subject-object condition is synonymous with ordinary mind, the ordinary mind is also dissolved. The answer to your question is that there is neither one who knows or that which is known. There is only Universal Mind, Unconditioned Intelligence, Pure Consciousness, Self.

Another Student: You say that the Self—or what I would call "God"—is pure Bliss, and I intuitively know that this is true. But isn't ordinary mind a projection of God? I mean, if ordinary mind is responsible for our suffering, why did it come into existence?

RH: You are dreaming that it exists. See if it really exists. Investigate.

Student: But I am speaking to you now, so I must be speaking the thoughts that come into my mind.

RH: Find out where your thoughts come from. See if you have a mind. You believe that "thoughts" travel through a "mind" like a train travels through a tunnel. These are illusions. They appear real like an illusion appears to be real. When the conjurer turns the rope into a snake, you say that you see the snake but you *know* it is really an illusion. When the snake is returned to its original form as a rope, you say, "I knew it was the rope all along." When the sun rises, do you say, "Where has the darkness gone?" No, the darkness is simply the absence of light. In the same way, the illusion that you are a body and mind existing in a world disappears with the recognition of Self.

Student: Then you literally "lose your mind"?

RH: Nothing is lost. What is illusory cannot be lost.

Student: And you can continue to function?

RH: You see the power of ordinary mind? Even now it forces you to be concerned with illusion rather than Reality. You are more interested in discussing your bondage than your liberation. Students are always astonished when they first learn from the Yoga teachings that the ordinary mind and the world it projects are illusions. But, as they continue to practice, they become even *more* astonished that they once considered these things *real*!

Also, when some students first hear this doctrine—that the world is unreal in the Ultimate sense we have been discussing here—they begin to think of different ways to change the world or to eliminate it through what they think of as the "power of mind." But such efforts are futile and only increase their disturbance. They do not understand that it is necessary to find the *source* of the illusion by diving down to the *root* of the mind, to that place from where it arises.

Student: I feel perfectly contented with my life. I'm very happily married and have a lovely home and three children. I don't think I am suffering. I'm attending the workshop here to participate in the Hatha classes. I have a few physical problems I'm trying to overcome, that's all.

RH: That's fine. You will be helped by the Hatha classes. There is no reason for you to continue in these discussion groups. I suggest you go down to the beach and enjoy the sunshine we have today.

(This student left the hall.)

Another Student: Wouldn't she have benefitted by staying?

RH: She wanted to go. There is no value in detaining her.

Student: Do you think that she is *unconsciously* seeking?

RH: All are seeking. Now she seeks her fulfillment externally. When the time is ripe she will "awaken" and her consciousness will turn inward.

Another Student: I notice that you are now using the words *time* and *consciousness*. Don't these words imply that there is a "mind"?

RH: First, be aware of the fact that words are a most unsatisfactory medium to express the nature of the world and Self. In effect, we are attempting to describe the UNLIMITED with the limited. I have explained, however, that these words which often make the Yoga teachings appear ambiguous and contradictory are necessary for purposes of discussion and oral instruction. An infinitely more effective form of instruction and learning is silence. Meditation occurs in silence. I explain the nature of maya and of the mayic condition by utilizing the illusionary concepts of "mind", which include those of "time" and "space." My principal objective in all of this is not to exercise the mind and precipitate endless discussion. It is to convince you of the efficacy of meditation. All "progress" in your quest for Self is accomplished in meditation, both active and passive. So I use many devices to push you into meditation. For example, I have just used the word *progress*. But now, in the next breath, I tell you that in Reality there is no "progress." You do not progress in recognition of Self. You ARE Self; you have always been Self and you can never be other than Self. If Self were something to acquire through one or another activity or effort, It could not be real and external; it could not be your true nature. How can you be apart from your true nature? So, with one breath I speak to you from the circumference of the circle and tell you about "progress"; with the next breath I speak to you from the center of the circle and tell you that in reality *there is no progress*. I vacillate between conditions as they appear in the mayic state (the circumference of the circle) and in the unconditioned nature of Self (the center of the circle). By going back and forth this way, at some point I will pull your ordinary mind inward toward the center. If I can pull you in for even a brief moment now and then, it will be an experience of the first magnitude for you. All doubts of the Truth of what I have been telling you are instantaneously dispelled. When you are pulled back by your ordinary mind to the circumference, the doubts will return. But they will return with less intensity. This back-and-forth process, coupled with serious meditation, will allow you to remain in the center for longer and longer intervals. The greatest wonder and mystery of all is that when you *are* in the center you realize that you have *always* been in the center, even when you dreamed you were on the circumference (in the world). From the circumference, you can envision the possibility of a center, as we have been discussing here. But from the center there is no circumference; indeed, there is no center! There is only Self.

Student: Are *you* always in the center?

RH: Of course, exactly as you are. There is no place else you can be.

Student: But do you always know it?

RH: Of course, exactly as you do. How can you not always Know the source of your existence?

Student: I don't always know it.

RH: Find out who it is that says he "doesn't know." The moment you find out, you will recognize that you are, and always have been, in the center.

Student: You frequently tell us to find out *"who* we are" and *"where* we are."

RH: Yes, these appear as two questions, but they are really the same. When you perceive *who* you are, you know from *where* the "I" arises, and, conversely, when you know *where* your "I" is, you know its nature, you understand how "you" are an invention of ordinary mind. So either question will lead you to the same point.

My teachings include the self-inquiry method of Ramana Maharshi. He was the great Indian saint and teacher of this century [1879–1950]. His principle technique was that of self-inquiry [*vichara*], which consists of the student's questioning of himself: "Who am I?" and/or "Where am I?" This forces a continual turning inward of the mind. People ask thousands of questions about things that are alien to their true natures, believing that the answers to these questions will eventually lead them to some extremely significant *truth*. But these answers only lead to more questions, without end. In reality there is only one question to be answered: "Who—or Where—am I?" The answer to this question will put an end to all other questions.

Student: Can *you* tell me where I am?

RH: Do you stand in your front yard and ask those who pass by on the street for directions to your house? They will tell you that you're already home.

Student: I find it very confusing to be somewhere and not know it!
  (Laughter)

RH: Abandon the ordinary-mind fantasies of "confusion" and "knowledge." These inventions of the ordinary mind have nothing to do with *you*.

Student: Then why am I confused?

RH: Find out *who* it is that is experiencing the confusion.

Another Student: How do you find out? How do you investigate?

RH: Yes, that is the pertinent question: "How?" I must say that as a group you have been a long time in asking it. The ordinary mind delays or avoids this question. It detects a major threat in the "Who?" and "Where?" investigation, which may lead to the exposure of its illusory nature. And what entity wishes to preside over its own dissolution?

The technique is this: During that time which you daily set aside for meditation, you silently ask yourself, "Where am I?" Now, this is a question which the computer, the ordinary mind, rejects as "illogical input." That is, it can respond at once with the present location of your physical organism. This response occurs from the mind being turned *outward* in its usual posture. But the physical location of the body is not the response we are seeking. We are attempting to determine whence the "I" arises. So we reintroduce the question "Where am I?" And the computer says, "I just told you. You are sitting here. . . ." And so you introduce the question once again, and then again. You must be very attentive to the process and not allow the mind to lose its interest in the question and wander off to other matters. Each time you detect it wandering you must draw it back to the question. Eventually, that moment will come when the mind, exhausted by the constant reintroduction of the question, and unable to furnish the response that will enable it to free itself and resume its usual frantic motion, will turn *inward*. This moment represents a major development; from that point on, you can begin to Know.

Student: Isn't it possible for you to tell us directly where to look and save us the struggle involved in this process?

RH: No. There are no oral directions that "tell" the way. The "way" is seen in meditation; therefore, the process is indispensable.

Another Student: I know from experience that the mind is very difficult to control in these meditation practices.

RH: Of course. A horse that has gone unbridled for its entire life will vigorously resist any attempt at control. This is the situation with the ordinary mind. We can also liken it to a wild monkey that has been bitten by a swarm of bees. If you can imagine a creature in such a state of vexation, you can sense what the mind is like. It is this very uncontrolled wildness and agitation of the ordinary mind, in which it is turned continually outward and leaps about like the wretched monkey of which we just spoke, that binds you without respite to the external world and prevents you from knowing who and where you are. All attempts to change this pattern will meet with the most fierce resistance from ordinary mind. Beginning students of meditation are well aware of this resistance. Frequently, as the time for meditation practice approaches, they find that anything and everything suddenly assumes more importance. In this way, the ordinary mind desperately struggles to prevent its subjugation and eventual exposure. You must recognize its machinations and persevere in your practice.

Student: How long can it take for the mind to turn inward?

RH: No prediction can be made, nor is any necessary. In each person the condition of the consciousness, the state of ripeness, is different.

Another Student: I've never become serious about meditation, although I've tried it a few times. I know my mind is really wild and I think things would develop very slowly for me.

RH: You *don't* know this. All such speculations distract one from what must be accomplished. Begin to meditate seriously *now* and don't attempt to evaluate the state of your consciousness. Of what consequence is time? Meditation, active and passive, is the true business of our lives.

Another Student: Can the mind be turned inward and fixed there for a significant interval the first time one meditates?

RH: Certainly. But again, such speculations are of no value. These are more of the evasive and delaying tactics of ordinary mind.

Student: Suppose that I succeed in turning inward. How do I know what to do or where to go then?

RH: You will be guided, certainly from within, and possibly externally, by the appearance of a guide. The process of transformation that occurs from the inward turning of the ordinary mind is as natural as breathing. Do not be concerned. Just persist in your serious practice.

Student: Is ten or fifteen minutes daily sufficient time to devote?

RH: Begin with whatever is comfortable. Continue each session until you become fatigued. At first, the inquiry of "Where am I?"—or any other technique you're using—can be confined to that time when you sit down quietly once or twice daily. I refer to this as "passive" meditation. Gradually, however, you will find that the "seed" of your meditation—that is, what-

ever you have chosen for the meditation practice—
begins to manifest even when you are engaged in your
usual worldly activities. You begin to recognize that
meditation is your true nature and that you are always
in the meditative state.

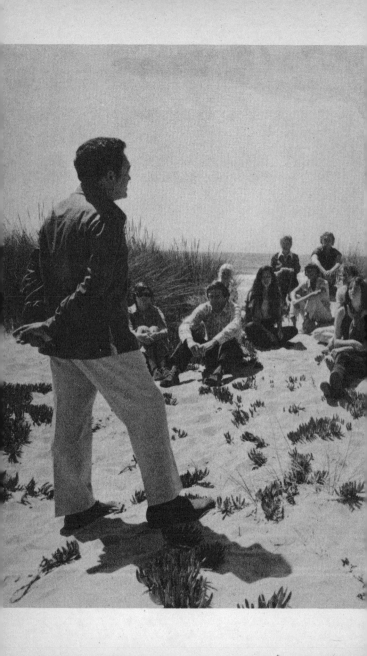

2nd day

Student: It seems that the entire meditation practice is involved with self and Self. This may be a foolish question, but doesn't this preoccupation with my self make me self-ish?

RH: First, let me say that I never consider any question which is concerned with one's freedom from bondage as "foolish."

One of the countless myths perpetrated by ordinary mind is that when you are involved with yourself you are "selfish," and when you are involved with others or are doing things for others you are somehow "unselfish." The truth is that if you do not manifest as Self you are totally selfish, regardless of what you are doing and how you wish to think about what you are doing. But manifesting Self, acting from the center, you cannot be selfish regardless of what you are doing.

Student: If I do volunteer service in helping the blind, how can that be considered selfish?

RH: Because it is done in the state of selfhood with the sense that *you* are the one who is volunteering and helping.

Student: Is that wrong?

RH: It is not a matter of right and wrong. No one is questioning your motives or telling you to withhold your services. You spoke of becoming "selfish" through the meditation—self-inquiry—I suggested, and so I tell you that all thoughts and actions emanating from the state of selfhood are self-ish. As such, the notion of "I am helping" is always present.

Student: I see what you're saying.

RH: Why do you volunteer your services?

Student: Because these blind people need help in various things.

RH: Examine the impulse which has moved you to volunteer. See where it comes from; trace it to its source. There you will discover *who* it is that is volunteering.

Another Student: Does one derive good karma from doing good deeds, from helping others?

RH: Yes . . .Why do you want good karma?

Student: I'm not sure.

RH: Then let us understand the real significance of "karma." There are three types of karma: that which is carried over into this incarnation from previous incarnations and which is discharged during this incarnation; that which is carried over from previous incarnations and is *not* discharged in this incarnation; that which is generated in this incarnation and, together with the second type, is carried over into future incarnations.

Karma is defined as "cause and effect," that is, as

the natural consequence of any particular thought or action. As such, *everything* that occurs can be explained as "karma." A person's karma consists of whatever he is presently experiencing or whatever he has yet to experience. These experiences are the results of actions that he has performed or is now performing. When a person is successful in a particular venture or when a pleasant experience befalls him, you may hear someone comment, "Oh, he must have good karma." Such a comment is meaningless; it explains nothing except that cause and effect are facts of the mayic condition, that action and reaction are inherent in the ego's existence.

But there is a more significant interpretation of "good karma." In the classical sense, good karma manifests as a force that guides the seeker into those auspicious situations where he has access to the teachings of Self-recognition. In India, for example, when one is born into a family where he will be exposed to the pure spiritual doctrines, he is said to have "good karma."

Student: Then bad karma has the opposite effect?

RH: Yes. Again, the superficial interpretation is that one who has accumulated bad karma will experience adversities in his worldly life. But classically, the meaning is that a person who has performed those actions which result in negative karma will have his recognition of Self seriously impeded. He will find it exceedingly difficult to overcome his ignorance and make progress in shaking off the bonds that tie him to the ego. Therefore, in this classical sense, one may appear highly "successful" in the way in which the conspirators evaluate "success" in the world, but yet may actually be experiencing bad karma. If his "success," "wealth," or whatever, does not result in his "awakening" to his real condition in maya, in his becoming a seeker, of what value is it? That is why Jesus said, "It is easier for a camel to pass through the eye of a needle than for a rich man . . ." Conversely, a person whose worldly life is difficult, and whom you may characterize as having "bad karma," may, exactly *because* of these difficulties, be led to search for the cause of his hardships. This search can result in his "awakening." So the man who has an insight into the nature of karma is actually reluctant to use the word at all.

Another Student: You're always hearing about the doctrine of karma in relation to the Eastern religions and philosophies. Why is it so important there?

RH: For several reasons. For those whose capacity to understand the pure doctrine is not sufficiently developed, karma acts as a doctrine of morality. It teaches, "As you sow, so shall you reap," and this teaching is understood and applied on the gross level. One is thus inclined to walk the "straight and narrow."

Next, in the more highly evolved Eastern religions and philosophies, the doctrine of karma assists the adherents in understanding that life is not the incomprehensible creation of an entity which bestows favors and takes revenge according to some unfathomable reasoning, but that effects are the result of the thoughts and actions of the individual man and woman. Here, karma imparts a type of "scientific" perspective to life; one is somewhat aware that justice and punishment lie in his own hands.

Finally, for those who are more highly evolved, karma serves as the doctrine that continually reinforces the desirability of liberation from the ego. The reasoning is this: each cause (action, thought) has an effect (result). These effects can be the immediate results of an action or thought, but they can also be delayed— delayed in terms not only of months or years but of lifetimes. That is, if the physical body does not live long enough for the effects to manifest, these effects do not dissolve with the death of the body; they remain in a latent state. But because they *must* manifest, at the propitious moment the ego assumes a new body; which makes their manifestation possible. However, you must understand that *new* thoughts and *new* actions are generating new karma each moment. Because new karma is endless, the necessity for a new body, for another cycle of birth and death, must be endless. How will this cycle be terminated? Only by the annihilation of the ego. This annihilation is accomplished by mergence with Self (Yoga). So, with this doctrine of karma always in the background, the seeker is moved to sustain his serious efforts for liberation from the cycle of birth and death.

Another Student: If one has good karma in the sense you have defined it, how does this manifest in death?

RH: The scriptures state that the plane [*loka*] where the ego abides when it is not incarnate is in accordance with the karma it has garnered during the incarnation. "Wrong" actions result in bad karma, which has its unhappy consequences. "Right" actions result in good karma, which has its happy consequences. When each has expired, rebirth occurs. The entire process then repeats. So for those who seek liberation, of what value is either good or bad karma?

Student: Can one know one's past incarnations?

RH: It is possible. But again, why waste your time in such endeavors? You must find out *who* you are in *this* incarnation. Remember, it is the ego that incarnates. It is the ego that projects the body and the universe. You think that you are in the universe, but the Truth is that the universe is in you.

Another Student: I would like to know what the scriptures which you just mentioned regard as "good" karma.

RH: Service, devotion to God or Brahma, self-surrender. But I trust I've made it very clear that any intentional efforts to accumulate "good" karma are for those who are unable to undertake the practice that results in the *direct* recognition of Self. Right action and good karma comprise the *indirect* path that leads to the eventual recognition of Self. Certain methods of meditation, including self-inquiry, lead to *direct* annihilation of the ego. The ultimate effect of good karma is your exposure to the pure doctrine. But you are hearing that doctrine here and now. So why plan for a future time or for future lifetimes? Manifest Self NOW.

Student: The *Bhagavad-Gita* tells us that "All eventually come unto Me." This means, I assume, that everyone will attain Self. Is that correct?

RH: Yes. All who do not recognize that they ARE SELF will "attain" SELF.

Student: Then why should we undertake meditations or any such practices at all?

RH: How long is "eventually"? When one begins to have an insight into the condition in the mayic state and the endless suffering caused by his identification with the ego, the principal business of his life becomes liberation *now*. He has no wish to suffer through countless future lifetimes.

Another Student: What if one doesn't believe in reincarnation?

RH: If you have only this lifetime, then that is all the more reason to dedicate yourself fully to the work at hand. Enlightenment will not come without effort. Your next breath may be your last of this incarnation, so do not delay your efforts.

Another Student: Men such as Krishnamurti and Alan Watts have written that effort is unnecessary, that all we need to do is be ourselves.

RH: Not "be yourself." Only BE . . .Do you understand this?

Student (After a pause): No, not fully.

RH: Then effort is necessary. It is necessary until Self-consciousness is restored. Only then will you comprehend that effort has not been necessary.

Student: How peculiar!

RH: Peculiar and enigmatic from the circumference of the circle; peculiar for the ordinary mind, which cannot deal with such illogical input. But not peculiar for Self, which encompasses all and IS ALL.

Student: Alan Watts mentions you in his autobiography, which I just finished reading.

RH: I had many good times with Alan when he was dean of the American Academy of Asian Studies in San Francisco. That was about twenty years ago.

Student: Do you think he was an enlightened man?

RH: All are enlightened; it is only necessary to recognize the Reality of your enlightenment.

Another Student: The Taoists say that you must "get out of your own way."

RH: That's another way of putting it. The ego, the I, is what is in your way. When its illusory nature is exposed, it dissolves.

Previous Student: But what I meant about Watts is that he seemed so completely set against meditation and similar practices, and I'm trying to evaluate that in light of what we've been discussing here.

RH: Don't concern yourself with "evaluation." It is not within the province of your ordinary mind to make a *decision* as to whether or not to meditate. If you begin to awaken from the dream of the ego, from the dream of confinement in a body and mind, a force that is far more powerful than ordinary mind will eventually compel you to undertake the necessary practices. Try as it may, your ordinary mind will ultimately be unable to obstruct your journey to Self-recognition, whatever the form that this journey takes. "Evaluation" is an exercise for the ordinary mind. Self does not evaluate.

Another Student: Then that person whom you refer to as "awakened" will not go back to sleep?

RH: No. Once having awakened, you become a seeker. You may rest and you may even nap, but you cannot lapse back into your former deep sleep. You are compelled to move forward. From time to time your path will be obscured, and occasionally you will feel that you are taking some backward steps. Obstacles will be encountered. But all will be overcome; there can be no doubt as to the outcome.

Another Student: It's certainly comforting to hear you say that, because when you're in the midst of those obstacles you sure can't see the light and you're inclined to back off and forget the whole thing.

RH: You already know that it is not possible to "forget the whole thing." Your business in this life is to remember *who you are*. There can be no "backing off" from this.

Another Student: I want to be sure I understand something here. We are now speaking of "being asleep" as opposed to "being awake," and we are also talking about "obstacles," about "moving forward and backward." But actually, none of these things or states are real. Correct?

RH: Self is REAL. Self is ALL. That there is ignorance, that one can "awaken" from this ignorance, and that one can encounter "obstacles" during a "journey" on a "path" are all illusions. We utilize these illusions because they are concepts which the ordinary mind can grasp and consider. In its consideration of such things it will, at some point, be forced to turn inward. The mind is illuminated by this inward turning and this illumination is our objective. Illumination dispels darkness and dissolves illusions. In this way, we use the mind to transform and consume itself. The scriptures give the example of the stick that is used to stir the funeral pyre. In the course of the stirring, the stick is itself ignited and consumed. In the course of investigating itself through the meditative techniques we have suggested, the ordinary mind is consumed by the light of Self.

Student: So, although you refer to us as "seekers", there is really nothing to seek.

RH: Exactly so. There is always this ambiguity when one

attempts to indicate the UNLIMITED (Self) with the limited (words). You are drawn to Yoga practice because you are looking for something; you have an objective. In this sense you are a seeker. When you recognize that your practice is your objective, that *the practice becomes the goal*, you will cease to be a seeker. Ultimately, you understand that you have never sought because there is nothing to seek. Self is your true nature and you can never be other than Self.

Student: But now, at this time, even if I know that there is nothing to seek, I still must seek.

RH: Yes, because you are saying you "know" with your intellect. You are thinking of "knowing" as the opposite of "not knowing," of being ignorant. You believe you can perceive your true nature through the accumulation of knowledge. But when one is occupied with knowledge, wisdom is excluded. Relinquish these creations of the intellect and you will truly Know.

Another Student: Then it is pointless for me to believe I have awakened and that I am a seeker on a path, for there is really no awakening and no path!

RH: Do you say this from your awareness of Self, or is it proceeding from the intellect?

Student (After a pause): I don't know. I'm trying to feel.

RH: If you don't know, then you must continue as a seeker on your path. You are always free to manifest Self and terminate your seeking.

Student: Do all the major religions in the world teach the way to Self?

RH: All proclaim the fact of Self as God, Brahma, and so forth. Most also recognize the need for ego annihilation. However, the methods that are advanced for ego annihilation and Self-recognition are, in many of these religions, what I refer to as "indirect."

Student: Can you give us some examples?

RH: It's unnecessary. We have no need to refute, or contend, or become enmeshed in controversy.

Student: But I would like to be able to present your viewpoint on a number of these religious matters in discussions I have with certain people.

RH: I advise against such discussions. They are pointless and enervating. Practicing Yogis do not expend their energies in these types of discussions.

Student: Don't you think it's helpful to others if you can point out genuine fallacies in some of the things they believe in with all their hearts? I mean, if you can do it sincerely and without offending them?

RH: What business is it of yours what others believe in? You should first find out what *you* believe in. You believe that you are contained within a body and a mind. See if *this* belief is valid. Then you will know if it is necessary for you to instruct others and change their beliefs.

Student: You are instructing us. You are changing *our* beliefs.

RH: It is not my intention to do so. I have no interest in "beliefs." I teach only the fact of Self. If such instruction causes your ordinary mind to substitute one illusion for another—that is, one belief for another—my instruction is indirect.

Student: You have taught me to believe in Self.

RH: Are you two selves—one that "believes" in another? Self is not to be believed in. Self IS.

Another Student: You frequently use the word *recognize* in relation to Self. Do you think that's the best word?

RH: Well, *recognize* means to "know again." It may come close to indicating that state at which we are pointing a finger. Obviously no word is adequate, but I prefer *recognize* to *realization*. I also use other words such as *awareness* and *manifest* according to what a particular explanation may seem to warrant.

Student: I notice that you just used the word *prefer*. Do you have preferences?

RH: One can make choices and indicate distinctions without having preferences in the sense in which "preference" is usually understood. In all such distinctions it is the absence of the "I" that is critical. The state of Enlightenment is sometimes defined as "choiceless awareness." The enlightened man may appear to choose, but the absence of ego nullifies the karma which is accumulated by the ordinary man in *his* choosing.

Another Student: I would like to get back to religion for a moment. If one is a Catholic or Jew and becomes interested in Yoga and the Yoga philosophy, how can one become actively involved in the Yoga practices? I mean how can the doctrines be reconciled?

RH: You are assuming that these doctrines are in conflict. I see no conflict. At one time, in my ignorance, I did distinguish among them. But as my understanding and insight increased, the conflicts were resolved and eventually disappeared. Moses, David, Solomon, the prophets, Christ and other gurus of the Old and New Testaments, these were great saints and Yogis. They incarnated as guides to Self. They instructed those who had "eyes to see" and "ears to hear." Moses, Gautama, Jesus, Mohammed, Ramakrishna, and Maharshi taught the Self-doctrine to different people at different times and in varying situations. Therefore, there may appear to be differences among their teachings. But these are superficial. They all taught from Self. If you view their teachings with this knowledge, there is no contradiction or conflict. There is only Self. Self is devoid of differentiation. The superficial distinctions of the teachings have been accentuated through misinterpretations by those who came afterward and who did not possess the pure Knowledge of Self. The blind led the blind: the distinctions became the bases for all manner of doctrinal structures around which multitudes of peoples were organized. This process is ongoing: even today thousands are regularly slaughtered in "religious" wars. What has all this to do with Self?

Student: So one who seeks Self in the pure or direct way cannot be part of an organized religion.

RH: That is not necessarily true. Each person will make that determination according to his or her level of understanding. If you recognize that the true basis of your religion is in Self, there may be no need to abandon this religion; only the perspective will change.

Student: But it does seem to me that if I undertook the Yoga practice seriously I could not continue to subscribe to certain tenets of my religion regarding the nature of God and His actions, and I could not continue to worship in the same way as I have in the past.

RH: There is no need for you to make a decision about this now. As your understanding increases, certain changes will evolve naturally. These will be recognized as the natural course of development and you will not feel that you are forsaking or renouncing your religion. When one grows from youth to middle-age, one does not feel that he has betrayed his childhood. The development is entirely natural. In the same way, your growth in Self-awareness is natural. However, if a sense of conflict should remain, you will always find the way to incorporate this growth into the existing structure of the religion. This incorporation of new interpretations into their religions has been the accomplishment of many outstanding religious leaders.

Student: But in order for this "growth" to materialize, do I not have to practice the Yoga techniques that we are learning here?

RH: The way you are learning Hatha Yoga here cannot be in conflict with any major religion. Nor can observation of the breath, quieting of the mind, self-inquiry, fixation of the attention upon a particular object, or listening for the inner sound be contrary to any liturgy. No deity, worship, ritual, ceremony, or prayer need be involved in your Yoga practice at this time. Of whom do you think the Yoga classes in the Western world are composed? There are very few Hindus and Buddhists. Primarily, these classes are made up of people who have a religion: Roman Catholics, orthodox Jews, Mormons, and probably just about any other you can name. Yoga presents the doctrine of Self; it seeks no converts.

Another Student: What about sin? I mean, the fact of sin is fundamental in most of Christianity and Judaism.

RH: All sin is ignorance of Self. There is no "fact of sin" in Self.

Student: The entire basis of Christianity is sin and redemption.

RH: The teachings of those around whom the religions have been structured are primarily concerned with recognition of Self. Attain Self and then you will know about "sin and redemption." "Seek first the kindgom of God."

Student: We are told that the original sin is desire for knowledge.

RH: Determine the *source* of this desire; relinquish your preoccupation with sin.

Another Student: Isn't murder a sin?

RH: Self cannot murder.

Student: But if a man murders another, has he not committed a sin?

RH: What will it profit you to know if murder is a sin or not? Will you consider murder permissible if I say that it is not a sin? Are you planning to murder someone?
(Laughter)

Student: No. At least not at the present time.

RH: Then attend to your practice and don't be concerned about who may murder whom. These are endless speculations of the ordinary mind. They distract you from turning the mind inward.

Student: All right. But let me ask just one more thing on this subject. If I see a man about to harm another man, shouldn't I prevent him? Shouldn't I be concerned?

RH: When that situation arises, you will act as you must. All these anticipations and fantasies of how one should act in a particular situation turn you away from Self.

Another Student: My work brings me into contact with many religious leaders. Very few of these seem to me to be people who have achieved Self-consciousness.

RH: In what way does this concern you?

Student: Well, I mean just personally, when I go into a church and listen to the sermon, it's obvious to me that the reverend who is delivering the sermon has not transcended his ego, and the sermon is meaningless; often it's ridiculous.

RH: Then why do you attend?

Student: It's expected of me.

RH: You must recognize that those who are in attendance at that sermon are also seeking. Their level of understanding may not be as yours, but, nonetheless, they are seeking, and that very sermon may be quite meaningful to many among them. Those who have not had your opportunities deserve your tolerance and compassion. Recognize everyone as seeking Self—the learned and the unlearned.

Student: It is certainly difficult to understand how many of the people that you see in everyday life are seeking the spiritual experience.

RH: Jesus taught that first the mote was to be cast from one's own eye. This is not to be understood in the superficial sense that each has his own personality flaws, but rather that, in ceasing to judge and in turning the mind inward, there is no possibility of perceiving faults and errors in other people; indeed, when you recognize that you have no self, then there are no "others" to be judged!

RH: Man's condition in maya is indeed wondrous. He will happily run to the ends of the earth to acquire and possess something and he will thank you for sending him there. But if you tell him that he now possesses infinitely more than he can ever hope to acquire, he will become resentful and tell you to leave him alone.

Student: Because he can't imagine it's true.

RH: That's the gist of it. . . . But then there is one who, when he hears that he already has what he has been searching for, says to himself, "Yes, I see. I have been looking in the wrong direction. The treasure is within. I must look within." Why does this man hear and understand, and the others do not?

Student: He must be ripe and have "ears to hear."

RH: Yes. The teachings of the wise men are certainly like seeds that are cast about the countryside. Only those seeds that fall into fertile soil will take root and grow. So it is that only one man out of many is prepared to receive the teachings and nurture them.

Another Student: He must have the type of good karma we were talking about.

RH: That is an acceptable explanation. In many of the Eastern philosophies this condition is also characterized as "having received grace." That is, his heart and intellect have been made receptive. It is similar to what we understand as "grace" in Christianity. The system that is primarily concerned with the practitioner's active seeking of grace is Bhakti Yoga. The Bhakta [devotee] is of service to the community and the society, and practices *self-surrender*. Bhakti is the most simple of the Yogas and was pronounced as "fit for all" by the ancients. Anyone who is strongly inclined toward being of help to others, or who has an innate love for nature, for his fellow man, for animals, is particularly suited for the practice of Bhakti.

The principal practice of the Bhakta is that of self-surrender. He is always permeated with the thought, "Not I, but Thou." Whatever his actions and the fruits of these actions, he dedicates them to the Lord. This is his path to self-effacement, to the dissolution of the ego.

Student: And Self can be attained this way?

RH: The only obstacle to uncovering Self is the illusion of self, of mistaking the not real for the Real. Remove this ego illusion and there remains only Self. So the Bhakta is saying, "Lord, help me to Know that there is only You. I dedicate all to You. I am not responsible for my life because I place it entirely in Your hands. *You* are the doer; I am a vessel through which you manifest." In this manner the Bhakta seeks Self.

Student: But unless divine intervention is a fact, then what you just said is again ordinary mind petitioning ordinary mind. Ordinary mind is asking ordinary mind to efface itself.

RH: It can be viewed that way. We have spoken of the value of turning ordinary mind upon itself so that it is ultimately pulled inward to Self.

Another Student: The words *outward* and *inward* still confuse me.

RH: There is neither inward or outward in Reality. We use the word *inward* in our discussions here to indicate a dimension other than that in which you identify with a body and mind which live in a world. We accommodate ordinary mind with the words *inward* and *outward*; these are things it can deal with. In effect, we attempt to move ordinary mind into a channel where it will be more and more subject to illumination.

Another Student: Do the body and mind and world *exist*?

RH: If by "existence" you mean the cognition of any thing through the senses, then the world and all in it may be said to "exist." But each thing is forever changing, simultaneously becoming and unbecoming. Nothing can remain constant for the least fraction of a second, so everything must be cognized *anew* every moment. Existence may appear to have a continuity, but if you look closely you must conclude that it arises spontaneously each instant. The fact that you can reach out your hand and touch this solid table and "feel" it does not mean it is not, along with everything else in this room, in a continual state of flux. You are inclined to equate what can be "sensed" with what is real. But where is its reality if it is *not* cognized by the senses? It is the senses and the thoughts, comprising the ordinary mind, that create the illusion of "reality." But if you attempt to grasp this reality, this existence, you find you cannot. It is an illusion; an illusion is unreal. You are Self. Self is eternally constant. It does not grow, decay, or die. There has never been a time when It was not, and there will never be a time when It will cease to Be. It simply IS. Therefore, only Self is Real.

Student: So can you say that *Self exists*?

RH: "Existence" and "non existence" are creations of the ordinary mind. Self transcends all such dualities.

Another Student: If Self is All, why does It permit the illusion of body, mind, and world to come into being?

RH: Find out if it has, indeed, "come into being."

Student: How?

RH: Turn the mind inward. When it is turned outward, the world appears. When it is turned inward, you discover where the world originates.

Student: Is the world thought?

RH: Yes, the world about which you are now speaking.

Student: Then the world can be influenced or changed by thought?

RH: Yes, the world that you project.

Student: You mean that different people project different worlds?

RH: Find out if there are "different people" who exist as realities and are apart from Self.

Another Student: What is the most effective way of influencing the world through thought?

RH: Why would you want to waste your time "influencing the world"? Do you want to transform one illusion into another?

(The student did not reply.)

Another Student: I think he's asking if the right kind of thought can improve conditions in the world.

RH: Who has created the world?

Student: I don't know.

RH: Then find out before you decide to improve it.

Another Student: God has created the world.

RH: Then allow God to take care of His creation. Do you presume to "improve" God's creation?

Student: It is our duty to improve it when and where we have the opportunity to do so.

RH: Does the world come to you and say, "Please improve me?" No. *You* have decided that the world needs improving. Your duty in life is to find out *Who you are.* Then you can improve the world if you wish.

Another Student: Are you saying that we are *not* to be of assistance to others when and where we can?

RH: Look how I am being attacked here on all sides!
(Laughter)
Isn't it fascinating how the ordinary mind makes you react—how indignant it has you become—when the altruistic role in which it casts you is being threatened? Ordinary mind convinces you that as bad,

evil, and rotten as you may be, you are, nonetheless, redeemed by the noble thoughts and actions of "relieving suffering" and "improving the world"!

You do not recognize the ingenuity of ordinary mind in keeping you continually off balance with these thoughts which effectively prevent you from turning inward. Again and again it is able to reinforce the illusion of its indispensability; in this case it is by telling you that it will direct you in "improving the world."

(Pause)

But to answer your question: Do whatever you must in any situation and do it to the fullest extent of your ability. But it must be done without any sense of "I." The thoughts "*I* am helping," "*I* am improving the world," and "*I* am alleviating suffering" must be transcended. In this way you will escape the karma that is generated if you believe *yourself* to be "improving the world."

Student: But that karma must be good.

RH: Good karma is not enlightenment and liberation.

Student: Are we not permitted to take satisfaction in doing good works and to enjoy their results?

RH: Ask yourself, "*Who* is it that wants to 'take satisfaction'?" If you discover *who* it is that is performing these good works and *who* it is that wants to "enjoy the results," your satisfaction and enjoyment will be beyond anything your ordinary mind has fantasized for you.

Student: Are those who have transcended the ego in the best position to be of service?

RH: They are not in any "position" at all. They are "of service" if that is what is to be done. Those who are expressing Self have no thought of "service" in the accepted sense of the word. They hold no thought of acting in order to be of service or to improve the world.

Student: Then why do they perform good works?

RH: Whatever their actions, they are *action-less*. They are ego-free.

Another Student: Was Gandhi such a person?

RH: Yes.

Student: How can you tell?

RH: By the manner in which he conducted his life.

Student: Why should it have befallen Gandhi to have to do what he did?

RH: It was the natural course of events. He had no sense of "having to do" anything. He did what came to him to do, just as *you* do what comes to you to do.

Student: Wasn't it his destiny?

RH: The word *destiny* is generally understood as the opposite of "free will." There is no such duality in Self. Self IS. Gandhi WAS. You must recognize that YOU ARE.

Another Student (After a pause): Would you say that Ghandi was free of karma during his life?

RH: It is pointless to speculate about such things. You must turn your attention to find out whether *you* are free of karma.

Student (Smiling): I don't think I am.

RH: Find out *who* it is that doesn't think so.

Another Student: You are always turning us upon ourselves.

RH: That is the instruction: turn the ordinary mind inward each time it wants to run away and perpetuate its illusions.

Student: You must get very tired of answering questions.

RH: That is the purpose of these meetings. Questions are asked about things that aren't known. What you don't know is endless; therefore, the questions are endless. The ordinary mind never reaches that point where it says, "There! That is the last question I need to ask. Now I know everything!"

(Laughter)

And, of course, what the ordinary mind does not know is endless, because it, itself, is continually and spontaneously creating an endless universe. You may believe that you are perceiving an external universe, an entity absolutely apart from you, and that the ingenuity and resourcefulness of the researchers in various fields will eventually enable you to know and understand all things about this universe. But the nature of the ordinary mind is such that it can never, in the ultimate sense, KNOW. It can create a universe and then appear to go in search of the "mysteries" of that universe. It gathers facts and statistics and it analyzes, evaluates, and performs all those functions of examination and investigation. It advances theories, which it then proceeds to change on a monthly or yearly basis as new evidence is "discovered." It speaks with authority on "man's problems," and it abstracts concepts of "God" and "God's plan." But it is really whistling in the dark about all of this. It can never Know because its nature is to remain in a perpetual subject-object relationship with that which it would Know. Each time it "solves" a problem, it is certain to create a multitude of additional problems. The problems thus become infinite. Amid all this problem making and problem solving, you are effectively diverted from recognizing your true nature, Self.

The value of the questions and answers in these meetings is that this ordinary-mind process may be exposed. We attempt to loosen the tentacles of ordinary mind by altering the way in which it is always flowing outward, by *interrupting* its outward flow. We dam it so that it must reverse its course and flow back toward its source.

Another Student: Many scientists and researchers are quite spiritual. They say that their work helps them to understand and appreciate the marvels of the Supreme Being. Some say that they have become religious as a result of their discoveries.

RH: We are not questioning the spirituality of scientists. I am suggesting that *you* examine the way in which *you* perceive the world, and trace your perception to its source. *Who* is it that sees the world?

Another Student: Getting back to Gandhi for a moment: he seemed to be a totally unique case. I mean, he *was* a politician and a leader, and such leaders are few and far between.

(Pause)

I was just making an observation. I guess I'm wondering why there aren't more politicians and leaders like he.

RH: Recognize that the world is always exactly as it must be. Once you lend credence to the thought that the world needs to be changed, when will such thoughts terminate? Will the world ever become as you desire it to be? If you believe that the world is a creation apart from you, let the Creator of the world take care of the world. Ramana Maharshi pointed out that when one rides on a bus or train he does not hold his luggage on his lap. He places it in the baggage compartment. If you believe you are existing—riding—in the world, then at least place the troubles of the world into the hands of the Creator. Don't carry them on your lap.

Student: It is extremely difficult not to want to change things.

RH: "Change" is the nature of the ordinary mind. You are Self and Self does not change.

Student: And you believe that Gandhi did not make a *conscious* observation that people were suffering and a *conscious* decision that he must do something about that suffering?

RH: His actions were rooted in Self. We need not speculate on his observations and decisions.

Student: Was he divinely guided in his actions?

RH: "Guidance" is for those who have yet to recognize that their true nature is Self. Once in the center, there is no longer any question of "success" and "failure," so there is no need for guidance.

Another Student: We really seem to want guidance in just about everything we do. We're afraid of being incorrect or making a wrong move.

RH: In the teaching of Yoga we urge the student to look more and more to himself for whatever guidance he feels is necessary in all matters. Such guidance is always forthcoming from within; you must learn how to listen for it with the inner ear.

Student: Is a guru [master] necessary?

RH: You already have your guru.

Student: I mean someone who would guide me personally on a continuing basis.

RH: I know what you mean. Don't you hear him guiding you?

Student: Are you referring to yourself?

RH: I am referring to the one who brought you here.

Student: I don't understand.

RH: You say you want "someone who can guide me." You identify with a body. Because you believe yourself encased in this physical organism, you look for a guru who also has a body. But the guru is within. It was the guru who awakened you, who has guided you since that time, and who has brought you here.

Student: I am not aware of this guidance.

RH: It is there like your heartbeat. Whenever you wish to become aware of your heartbeat you become still and direct your attention to it. In the same way, listen for the guru's instruction.

Another Student: How does he instruct?

RH: It cannot be described, but it is unmistakable.

Student: But it seems that we are able to communicate with a physical guru in a more direct and immediate way, like we are speaking to you here.

RH: And what will this physical guru do for you?

(The student did not reply.)

RH: He cannot impart enlightenment; he can only point the way. He points within and employs various devices to push you within. The real guidance comes from within. Why wait to be pushed? Turn inward now.

Another Student: The *shastras* [scriptures] say that association with a guru and with other enlightened people is essential for advancement.

RH: If and when the time comes that such associations are indispensable for you, they will materialize. There is not the slightest doubt of this. I tell you this so that you do not undertake the search for a physical guru with desperation, running here and there frantically, as so many are doing. This outward search has the effect of concealing from you the knowledge and certainty that the real guru lies within. In the outward search you can be distracted from your practice, from turning the mind inward. You may come to believe that unless you find a physical guru you cannot Be Self.

Student: Jesus said, "Seek and ye shall find."

RH: And you interpret this as pertaining to a guru? Why not interpret it as, "Seek and ye shall find fame and fortune"?

Student (After a pause): Yes, I suppose it can mean that whatever you seek you will find.

RH: In that case, seek and find Self, and all else will follow.

Student: Are you saying that no search whatsoever is required to find a guru?

RH: Trust the wisdom of the guru within. He knows if it is necessary for him to manifest in a physical form.

Student: Can you ask for instruction from the guru within?

RH: There is no need to ask. The instruction [*upadesa*] is always there. Learn to listen for it.

Another Student: Can you ask for guidance in a particular situation?

RH: There is no such thing as a "particular situation." All "situations" involve the outward flowing of the ordinary mind into an illusory, external world. The only guidance that will be given is to turn the mind inward and allow it to be drawn back into Self. Permit the "situations" to take care of themselves. Don't hold your luggage on your lap.

Student: But isn't this an avoidance of confronting life?

RH: In your delusion, you believe that you are an I, an ego, that maneuvers through the world, and that this ego is capable of "confronting" situations. In Reality, no such process occurs. The I does not act and cannot control or influence anything. Only recognize this and you will be spared the illusion of "confrontation."

Another Student: Hamlet agonized over whether to act or to withdraw. "To be or not to be," he said. "*That* is the question."

RH: In Reality, such a choice is not only unnecessary, it is impossible. His ignorance of this fact was the real reason for his agony. Neither to be nor not to be, *that* is the answer. Remain free from allying with one end of the stick and contriving to avoid the other end; duality [*dvaita*] is perpetual bondage.

Student: But life in the everyday world seems to entail the necessity of choices almost every minute.

RH: "Seems" is correct. In Truth, you do what you do *without* making a choice. It appears that the I is the chooser. Find out the nature of this I and you will discover that you act without choosing. *You are not the doer.*

Another Student: And if you are not the doer, then there is no karma from the action, right?

RH: Correct. You are free of both the action and the fruit of the action.

Another Student: I have been in group therapy for some years. The entire basis of the therapy is that by confronting those people and situations which disturb us, we learn how to deal with them and overcome them. This has been extremely helpful to me. I'm more confident and much more at ease in my life than I used to be.

RH: Yes, so?

Student: Well, I mean that if I hadn't taken a positive approach to my problems and learned how to confront things, I would have remained a much more troubled person.

RH What has all this to do with recognition of Self?

Student: I think that, being less disturbed, I am now in a position to practice Yoga, meditation, or whatever else I want to undertake.

RH: You are what you are at all times. If, at this point in your life, you undertake the practice of meditation, then such is the case. If at some previous time you thought you could not meditate because you were disturbed, then *that* was the case. No preliminaries are ever necessary to recognize that you are always Self. If your ordinary mind is able to convince you that it is necessary for you to engage in various preparations, that you must become more quiet, less disturbed, a better person, a "positive" thinker, more intelligent and so forth, then it has once again diverted you. You do not have to "improve" the ego in order to transcend it.

Student: But now that I recognize many of my "hang-ups," I know how to prevent my mind from getting "strung-out" with a lot of destructive stuff. I can usually catch myself before I go off in meaningless directions.

RH: All thoughts are destructive and all directions that you go off in are meaningless. All prevent you from turning inward.

(Pause)

Look at all the I's you are talking about. Which of these is the *real* I? Is it the one that you say "recognizes," or is it the one that has the "hang-ups"? Is it the one that "prevents," or is it the one that "goes off in directions"? And which is the I that can stand apart from all of these and tell us about them? Do you see that all this talk about what your different I's can do does not move you one iota closer to recognition of Self? Either you're immersed in your plurality of I's, or you perceive their nonexistence and you manifest Self.

Student: So you're saying that my knowing why I function as I do is of no help in achieving enlightenment?

RH: You *don't* know why you function as you do. You have only the continually changing concepts *about* your functioning that are presented to you by ordinary mind. Such concepts are not Knowledge. Self is Knowledge.

Student: And there's no value in understanding one's "hang-ups"?

RH: Get rid of both your "understanding" and your "hang-ups." Do you need to examine your garbage before you throw it out? If you undertake such examination, when will it end? The entity that is doing the examining is also manufacturing new garbage every moment.

Another Student: But if you are a tense person who is easily disturbed or if you are troubled with emotional problems it would be difficult to meditate.

RH: Is this ordinary-mind speculation or are you speaking from experience?

Student: Well, I haven't had too much experience.

RH: Then meditate first and make the statement afterward.

Another Student: Meditation, itself, helps you to eliminate tension and disturbances.

RH: Of course.

Another Student: What about people who are mentally deranged—can they practice meditation?

RH: Endless speculations! How will knowing this help you? Attend to your practice and then you can turn your attention to the deranged. Do you see how far afield ordinary mind leads you? Now you are concerned with the deranged, without understanding your own derangement. If you were not deranged, could you continually mistake the unreal for the Real? Would you remain in your prison cell when the door stands open for you to simply step outside to freedom? All those who languish in maya are deranged.

Student: Well, at least that explains it. I'm crazy.
(Laughter)

RH: Truly knowing that one is "crazy" to willingly remain in the burning house is an important step toward escape.

Student: You tell us to turn inward. What would become of society if everyone turned inward?

RH: This viewpoint is like that of the imprisoned man I was speaking of before. He has been told how to unlock the door of his cell and escape, but rather than dash to his freedom he is concerned with what would become of the prison if everyone in it escaped.

Student: But I have a family to take care of.

RH: Have you been told to abandon your family?

Student: No, but what if I lost interest in my job and my other commitments and my family suffered because of it?

RH: Do you feel you are being forced or coerced into understanding the nature of your existence in maya?

Student: No, not really. I guess I'm apprehensive about letting go of what I'm holding on to. I don't know where that would lead to. It's a sort of conflict I have.

RH: Where do you think you will be led? *You are now and always Self.* Ignorance of this Reality causes you to imagine yourself confined in a body and mind. Because this body moves about and changes its location, you believe that Self also moves. Self is unchanging, immutable. You cannot be "led" anywhere; wherever you think you go, you are, in Reality, always Self. You also believe that you can "hold on" to something or "let go" of it. In Reality, no such process transpires. You cannot "hold" Self and you cannot "let it go." Self IS.

[In a subsequent discussion, the student who asked the above questions was not present, but another man, who knew him personally, said that his friend had changed considerably since he had become interested in Yoga, about one year ago. When asked by another student to explain the nature of the "change," he replied that his friend seemed to be ambivalent, that he frequently expressed the desire to really "get into" Yoga, but that there was another part of him that was resisting. Mr. Hittleman made the following comments pertaining to this situation.]

RH: In the initial stages of what I designate "awakening," a person may experience illumination intermittently; the light comes and goes and the guru's instruction is, as yet heard only faintly. So, although he is drawn to and guided by the light, the awakened person is also still subject to the delusions of the sleeping man. Therefore, he has the feeling of being pulled in two directions simultaneously: toward the inner light and toward the world. This pulling frequently generates what is experienced as a "conflict," for all the obvious reasons. If we simply explain to the student that this conflict should be considered a natural development on the path, it can be helpful. If the student's capacity for understanding is adequate, we can advise that he direct his attention to the *source* of the conflict, to determining from *where* the conflict is arising.

Another Student: In Western mysticism this conflict is known as "purgation," the process of purification, so that one may know God. I mean, if we're speaking about "conflict" in the same sense.

RH: Yes. St. John of the Cross's "Dark Night of the Soul" is a beautiful expression of this viewpoint. However, "purification" is misleading. There is nothing to be purified. You are not an impure entity which requires purification before you can "know God." You need only abandon that which is of the not-Self and your purity will be evident.

Another Student: Certain religions would regard this as heresy.

RH: Because these religions teach that through purification one may become sufficiently cleansed of sin to *approach* God, but he can never become sufficiently purified to BE God! Approach—in an eternal subject-object relationship—is as far as man dare go. But, in Truth, All is Self; if All is Self can anything be apart from Self? Can *you* be apart from Self? No, you ARE Self. You and what you are conceiving as "God" are ONE. But man, in his ignorance, is conditioned to think otherwise.

[Because the above paragraphs were relevant to the man who was experiencing the "conflict," they were inserted at this point; actually, this conversation took place during the fourth day. The second day's discussion now continues.]

Student: Why does God create us and then obscure Himself from us?

RH: You are *assuming* that God has created us. It is *you* who are creating God. That which is "created" is subject to birth, growth, decay, and death. Your true nature does none of these things. Your ordinary mind creates God, Self, as an alternative to self, ego, I, and then pretends to go in "search" of its creation. But That which Self or God truly IS cannot be "known" by ordinary mind, for it transcends all those qualities by which the mind is able to "know." God is not lost in the sense that He needs to be "found." God, Self, is what you ARE. You need only put an end to what obscures this Reality. Therefore, let us leave God alone. Rather, examine your own existence. Do you deny your existence?

Student: No.

RH: Can you prove your existence to me?

Student: Well, I am here speaking with you.

RH: You say, "I am." Trace the source of that "I am." Find the point where it arises. Then you will know about God: whether He is hiding from you and whether He needs to be "found."

Student: I don't know where to look for that source.

RH: Do you mean that all day long you are saying, "I" this, and "I" that, and you don't know who that "I" is or where it comes from?

Student (After a pause): I am *me*.
   (The student then pointed to his chest and gave his name.)

RH: So your "I" is your name?

Student: Partially.

RH: And your "I" is your chest?

Student: Partially.

RH: And if we give you another name then that new name becomes your "I"?

(The student did not reply.)

RH: And when your chest or body dies, then your "I" dies?

Student: Do you mean the soul?

RH: So now you introduce another unknown element. Very well, I mean the soul. Does your soul die?

Student: I believe not. The soul does not die.

RH: So then there is something which you consider the essence of yourself, that is eternal, that does not die.

Student: I believe so.

RH: What is the nature of this "soul"?

Student: I don't know. It is subtle.

RH: Don't you find it extraordinary that you are ignorant of the nature of what you regard as the essence of your existence?

Student: Perhaps God does not wish us to know these things.

RH: Again "God"! Isn't the ordinary mind incredible? It presents a "God," of Whom it admittedly knows nothing, but Who is obscuring from us a "soul," of which it admittedly knows nothing, but which is the essence of an "I," which it locates in a transient body and mind. It would seem that you are existing in a peculiar state of ignorance about yourself.

(Pause)

Do you also see that within the next few minutes your ordinary mind can advance a multitude of "logical" reasons for this ignorance? A hundred arguments can be introduced. And as we discussed and debated each of these, you would be comfortably diverted from the reality of your basic ignorance: *you do not know your true nature.* That is why I always attempt to bring the ordinary mind back to this basic ignorance—to back it up against the wall and force it to acknowledge, without qualification, that it does not know the source of its origin, that it is a usurper of power, that it promises what it cannot fulfill: happiness, knowledge, peace. But it is as slippery as an eel. It squirms and writhes and wriggles out of such an acknowledgment and so we must catch it and push it up against the wall again and again. It will do anything to avoid our intensive scrutiny because it cannot survive such exposure. Among the numerous things it will invent, in order to escape investigation, are a "soul" and a "God." "God doesn't want us to know," you say, in final desperation. But we must persist; we persist until we are able to block all avenues of escape and the mind is forced to turn inward. That is the entire purpose of these discussions: not to exercise the ordinary mind and cater to its endless curiosities, but to confound or stun it long enough so that it will cease its outward flow and back up on itself, to maneuver it so that it has no alternative but to turn inward. Therefore, if at times I appear stern or uncompromising in response to your questions, you will understand that this is the posture that is required to bring the ordinary mind up short. Ordinary mind is the inventor of wild illusions and one suffers without end as long as its phantom nature remains unexposed.

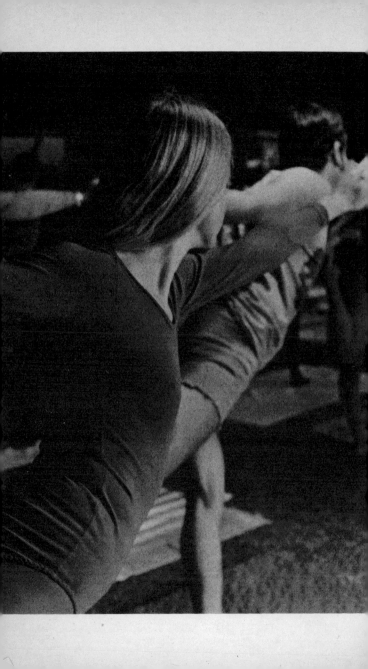

3rd day

Student: Mrs. F — — mentioned to me that she had a very severe headache this morning. She was experiencing a great deal of pain and she asked you what she could do for it, and you told her to lie down and you placed your hands on her head. She says that about fifteen minutes later the headache was gone and she felt fine. I'm very interested in faith healing and I wonder if you would speak about it.

RH: The word *faith* is misleading here. It implies that in doing whatever I did, I somehow became different from the way I usually am, that I assumed a different attitude or perspective. In other words, it implies that I am usually one way, and when I undertook to assist Mrs. F — — I petitioned some entity to give me added strength, power, or whatever. This was not the case.

Student: I think I understand. You just let the healing power flow through you.

RH: It is *always* flowing through you. You don't have to "let" it do anything. You simply need to BE. There is no "faith" involved in BEING. BEING is your true and only nature.

Student: All right. Then let me ask you about the techniques. When you placed your hands on her, what was in your mind? Or is it something else?

RH: When I do such things it is usually according to the "transference of the white light" technique. I have explained this fully in two of my books* and in a recording. One of the assistants here can give you the references.

Student: Does it always work?

RH: What do you mean by "work"?

Student: Does it always relieve the pain or cure the condition?

RH: We don't know. We can assume that in introducing this force, envisioned in the form of the white light, we increase the healing capacity of the organism. Some people experience immediate improvement, in others it is delayed, and in others there is no noticeable improvement even after a significant period of time has elapsed. I never anticipate results in these matters. That is, I introduce the white light and allow the organism to utilize it as it will. The wisdom of the body is to be trusted.

Also, I would comment on your use of the word *cure*. There is no "cure" involved in any method of natural healing, whether it be physical, "metaphysical," or nutritional. The organism simply returns to its natural state of health.

Student: What if it is an emergency? I mean, if someone is dying as the result of an injury.

Guide to Yoga Meditation and *Yoga: The 8 Steps to Health and Peace*

RH: The technique is the same. If the circumstances so indicate, I perform the white light transference.

Student: Must you have the person's cooperation?

RH: It is usually helpful, but not essential. However, you should not apply the technique if there is any resistance on the part of the intended recipient.

Student: Can this transference be performed from a distance? I mean, when you are not in physical contact with a person.

RH: Yes. The visualization is the same. During the exhalation, the hands may be extended straight outward and the light be directed toward the recipient, of whom you attempt to retain a mental image.

Student: I find that visualization which takes the form of seeing the ailing person in a state of total health is effective.

RH: Yes, that's good. There are many methods.

Another Student: There is something of Christian Science in a few of the remarks just made.

RH: Why must we classify? Will the technique be any more or less effective if it is classified?

Another Student: In what you said about "faith," it seemed to me that you discounted its value. Isn't faith important in all spiritual endeavors?

RH: Your nature is faith. You are always faith. You do not need to acquire it.

Student: But isn't it necessary to have faith that you will succeed in what you have undertaken, especially in a spiritual practice?

RH: It is more important to transcend your illusion of "succeeding" and "failing."

Student: When you encounter the various obstacles we were discussing, doesn't faith help strengthen your resolve to overcome them?

RH: This "faith" of which you are now speaking: how does it manifest? Do you have it at this moment?

Student: It's difficult to describe, but it seems to be something I reach out for, something like added force or belief.

RH: Where do you reach out for it?

Student: To something which is more powerful than myself.

RH: And is this "powerful" thing external to you? Is it somewhere in the world?

Student: No, it is within me.

RH: Precisely. You turn inward. You seek that "powerful" thing which transcends the ego. You wish to call it "faith," but you are really seeking to manifest Self. Faith *is* Self. There are no attributes or qualities apart from Self. So never mind about faith. Seek Self directly and all other things will follow. (This student was quiet for several moments. She had closed her eyes.)

Student (Smiling): Yes, yes. I see. It is all Self.

RH: Good. Remain there.

Another Student (Addressing the one who had just spoken): Can you tell us what you are now experiencing?

RH: If she attempts to describe it, it's gone.

Student: But once realizing Self, how can it be "gone"?

RH: Now you're on the right track. Self is not realized—made real—and it is not lost. However, the ordinary mind has held such a dominant position for so long that it can continue to reassert itself, so as to obscure Self. Therefore, one will usually experience being pulled out of the center by the ordinary mind and one must practice to continuously remember Self. The description you just requested from R—— reactivates her ordinary mind and pulls her from the center.

Student: So permanent recognition of Self is a *gradual* process?

RH: For most, it *appears* to be so. That ordinary mind can continue to reappear—although it does so with decreasing reality—is attributed to inclinations, tendencies, and predispositions [*vasanas*] that manifest as the result of actions performed in this and in previous incarnations. As I said, the strength of these tendencies diminishes with your serious meditation so that eventually their ability to pull you from the center is minimal.

But there are some who, experiencing Self for even an instant, remain as Self always. In these cases, the permanence is attributed to previous practice in past incarnations. The terms *gradual* and *sudden* are used only so that our instruction accommodates the ordinary mind.

Student: If the process is gradual—and I understand you are saying that the gradations seem real only from the circumference of the circle—then appealing to the intellect through discussion and reading can be helpful.

RH: Yes, providing such things are strictly limited and are accompanied by serious practice. A man who intellectually understands the nature of the sun knows that even when it is obscured by clouds it is still shining. He may say, "The sun isn't out today," but somewhere in himself he knows that it is *always* out. In the same way, our discussions help you to remember that *Self is always the Reality*, even when it appears to be obscured by ordinary mind. Just as one knows that by flying above the clouds the sun can always be seen, so should he know that by transcending the ordinary mind at any given moment, Self always IS.

Another Student: Doesn't it require faith to know that I am always Self?

RH: If your heart stops beating, the body will die. The heartbeat is a vital function and must continue each second. Since your life is dependent on your heartbeat, do you say, "I must have faith that my heart will continue to beat"?

Student: I seldom think about it.

RH: Yes. With or without your faith, your heartbeat goes on. How much more does Self continue as Reality, with or without your faith!

(Pause)

Do you understand? I am telling you that when you are sitting in your living room, all preparations to go home are unnecessary. Recognize that you are already home. When you go to the movies, do you take along a flashlight to see the screen? No. All the necessary illumination is forthcoming from the projector. In the same way, your faith, prayers, good deeds, and so forth are superfluous. All the illumination you require is emanating from Self.

Student: For several months I have been fixing my consciousness in the Ajna chakra during meditation. [The Ajna chakra is that subtle center located in the area between the eyebrows and sometimes referred to as the "third eye." It is the highest of the six chakras.] Recently, I've begun to have vivid visions of colored lights. They are beautiful and brilliant, brighter than anything I've ever seen with the physical eye, and they come and go in . . .waves. The colors are mostly those of the dark part of the spectrum: purple, green, and so forth. Can you comment on this?

RH: As the various chakras are "activated" through meditation, many such phenomena occur. *Who* sees these visions?

Student: Well . . .*I* do.

RH: So always there is a witness. Rather than be swept into these phenomena, you must continue to ask, "*Who* is the witness of these things?"

Student (After a pause): I understand. But, you know, when these lights appear they are so compelling that I want to observe them as long as they last. It is really difficult to think of anything else, I mean, to fix the consciousness elsewhere.

RH: All such phenomena, including whatever "powers" [*siddhis*] and so-called extrasensory perception manifest, must be regarded with dispassion. Certain Yoga scriptures describe them as "signposts along the path." They indicate that the inward journey is proceeding. However, the student is cautioned in the strongest terms against becoming involved with these visions and powers. Utilization of these powers can have the most adverse effect on the student's development. Always attempt to determine *who* it is that is experiencing the phenomena.

Another Student: There must be millions of people in the world who are attempting to cultivate ESP. You're always hearing about it everywhere.

RH: Because this "perception" is of a subtle nature, and the ordinary man is functioning on the gross plane, it is not *consciously* known to him. Therefore, he speaks of this unfamiliar level of perception as "extra." When the gross, outward-flowing senses which cognize the external world are turned inward, they become subtle. Clairvoyance, for example, is external sight turned inward. In addition to this subtle, "extra" perception, there are phenomena which exceed the ordinary man's wildest fantasies of power, control, and manipulation. None of these things are truly "extra" to the human being. They are wholly contained within the universe, the microcosm, of each person. To most, however, they remain "unknown."

During the course of Yoga and related practices, these subtle planes [*lokas*] are uncovered. The Yogi can explore and absorb them [*laya*] and utilize the elements of which they are composed. However, it is only the ill-advised student who will have the desire to involve himself with these elements for gratification. The ignorant man is highly desirous of uncovering, cultivating, and utilizing such powers because through them he envisions himself controlling, influencing, and manipulating people and conditions. But he desires all this exactly because he *is* ignorant. He has no comprehension that such powers are utterly useless in effecting his enlightenment and liberation; indeed, how can he understand what formidable *obstacles* they represent? He is unaware of seeking Self. If the doctrine of Self is explained to him, he has not "ears to hear." He remains asleep, dreaming of power, control, and manipulation to gratify his senses and ego in an illusory world. To him, such power may lie in ESP. So, although asleep to his real nature, he attempts to cultivate "powers."

The Yogi, the awakened man, understands the nature of his quest. He recognizes that Self manifests when he discards, eliminates, and transcends all that is of the not-Self. If he consciously seeks to accomplish anything, it is not to acquire, but to discard. Any need to cultivate ESP is totally absent. All desire to influence people and events, on whatever plane, and no matter how noble the motives or objectives, binds one to the not-Self, thereby perpetuating suffering. So shun the acquisition of power, influence, and control as you would the plague.

Another Student: But ESP properly applied could be used to the great benefit of mankind.

RH: That is a speculation of ordinary mind. First, find out what inhibits *your* fusion with Self. BE Self, then you can determine if mankind needs to be "benefitted."

Another Student: Before, when discussing some things about religion, you indicated that we *could* listen for the inner sound, look for the inner light, and so forth. Now you are telling us in no uncertain terms *not* to become involved in these things. This seems a direct contradiction.

RH: Listening for the inner sound, observing the breath, and all such practices are primarily for the purpose of aiding the mind in withdrawal from the external world and fixing the attention on a single point. In this way, you achieve one-pointedness. It is only when the mind is held fixed, steady and quiet, that one may perceive its nature. These practices have nothing whatsoever to do with the desire for developing ESP.

Student: There's one other thing. I believe it was on Monday that we were discussing mantras and you said that our name was an acceptable mantra because it was permeated with our essence. But a short while ago you said that the "I" was *not* in our name.

RH: Your "I" is your ego, not your essence. Dive deep within and find out what and where your "essence" is. The mantra helps to steady your mind and pull you inward.

Another Student: We were discussing "visions." Western religion and metaphysics are replete with examples of seekers who earnestly, even fanatically, sought visions.

RH: Such desires are obstacles. Visions are diversionary.

Student: They were yearning to see God.

RH: "God" and "Self" are conceptualized as the alternative to "self," to "ego." Put an end to conceptualization and there is no further need to "see God." The sufferings inherent in such yearnings are, indeed, *self*-inflicted.

Student: What about those who see Christ, the Virgin Mary, and the saints?

RH: Possible signs along the path. Observe them dispassionately and move along.

Student: A vision of Christ is said to evoke tremendous outpourings of love.

RH: Then pour out your love and move along.

Student: Is Christ Self?

RH: Yes. Christ told you that *All are Self.*

Student: Can Christ lead you to Self?

RH: Nothing "leads" to Self. Self IS.

Student: But you speak of a "path." Cannot Christ guide one on the path?

RH: Christ said, "I and my Father are One." If you are of a worshipful or Bhakti nature, then surrender your self—which is the not-Self—and all that can remain is Self. Complete surrender is what is required. If it helps you to surrender to Christ, then do so.

Student: And He will guide?

RH: He will do what He will. If you surrender, it must be absolute and unqualified. You cannot qualify your surrender with questions and petitions. When the Bhakta surrenders, he assumes no further responsibility for his life. It has been placed totally in the hands of the One to whom he has surrendered. Complete surrender, the path of Bhakti Yoga, is an alternative to the recognition of Self through the practices we are discussing: Kundalini, Jnana [self-inquiry], Raja.

Student: Do you recommend reading the Bible?

RH: If you read the Bible—or any scripture—from the viewpoint we have been advancing here, you will discern those sections which deal *directly* with the recognition of Self, and those which are *indirect*.

Another Student: You said to "end conceptualization." Is this the same as turning the ordinary mind inward?

RH: Yes. The "I" thought is the root of all thoughts. All thoughts arise from the concept of "I." Turn the mind inward and dive down to this root. When you cut out the root, you eliminate conceptualization.

Student: Are there such things as demons, evil spirits, and so forth?

RH: Have you seen them?

Student: I believe so.

RH: As with all phenomena, you should determine *who* is seeing them. Find out *where* they are originating.

Student: Can a spirit enter and take posession of one's body?

RH: You are asking if one illusion can possess another. Why do you trouble yourself with such things?

Student: Because I once had a drug experience during which I was certain that a lower spirit possessed me. I felt its influence for many days. It was a very negative, frightening experience and it was instrumental in turning me off of drugs, so I guess it was good in that respect. I don't even know how or why this spirit or whatever it was finally left, but it did.

RH: Always, in such experiences, you should question, "*Who* is being possessed? *Who* is experiencing the fear?" Through this questioning, these fantasies will be deprived of their power to disturb you and will cease to manifest.

Student: But you could be too frightened or distracted to do this.

RH: Practice always to turn the mind inward during all your activities. It will become easier and easier. Whenever you recognize that you are being hypnotized by the not-Self, by events and conditions that are external to your true nature, reverse the flow of ordinary mind: turn inward. Don't permit yourself to be hypnotized by your activities in the world.

Student: If you are hypnotized, how can you *recognize* that you're hypnotized?

RH: Through your Yoga practice, the intervals of hypnosis are *interrupted* with increasing frequency. Soon, even a moment's interruption will "awaken" you and you will Self-remember. More and more you will remember to Self-remember.

Student: How do we know that Self is not an illusion?

RH: What do you envision as "Self"? How do you conceive "Self"?

Student (After a pause): I have no conception of it.

RH: Then how can you question its reality? Only something that is cognized can be questioned as to whether it is real or illusory.

Student (After a pause): I mean, can Self be just another idea of the ordinary mind?

RH: The "self" of which, and with which, you are now speaking *is* just another idea. Your self is imagining a Self; your illusion is imagining an illusion. SELF is not an idea. It is your true nature, your only Reality. Transcend the *creator* of the ideas, ordinary mind, and there is no further problem of illusion and reality. When duality is transcended, Self remains.

Another Student: Is Self a void?

RH: What is your understanding of "void"?

Student: Empty. Nothing.

RH: Self is neither empty nor full, yet it is simultaneously nothing and everything.

Student: So there is no point in attempting to visualize Self?

RH: There is no one that can stand apart from Self and "visualize" it. You ARE Self.
  (Pause)
  However, those who cannot jump directly into the center NOW, can, if they are strongly attracted to imagery, abstract an image—some form or representation—to which they surrender the I, the ego. Understand, however, that this is only a device for those who find it truly helpful. All such devices are for the purpose of fixing the ordinary mind upon one point and holding it there. Those whose awareness is more developed will, rather, seek to know from *where* the visualization proceeds. They will look directly to the source.

Another Student: Does my mind function independently of what I refer to as "myself"? Sometimes it seems that I can stand back and watch my mind work.

RH: Ordinary mind is asking if it can stand back and watch itself. The seer and that which is seen are One. The thinker and that which is thought are One. Therefore, find out *who* is seeing and thinking, and you will awaken from the subject-object dream.

Student: Is mind an *agent* of Self? I mean, is it *within* Self?

RH: Your question implies a *whole* which is composed of *parts*. "The Self," you say, "has a mind within it." So you acknowledge multiplicity and, by so doing, are prevented from Knowing that Self is All. Self *is* the mind; Self *is* the projection; Self *is* the seer, the seen, and that means by which the seer sees the seen. *The eternal indivisibility of Self* is what must be recognized.

"I AM," said the Lord. Not, "I am a mind," and "I am the projection of a world," and "I am this and I am that." Only, "I AM." The creation and all that is known in the creation, and the uncreated and all that is unknown in the uncreated, are Real when this ONENESS is recognized. The moment the ONENESS is conceived as having any parts or qualities whatsoever, illusion manifests and all is unreal. SELF is real because of its indivisible Oneness. The self is illusory because of its multiplicity. The instant that a "second" arises, you are bound by the subject-object perception, you are a victim of the condition of duality.

Another Student (After an interval of silence): Why does the Self, the Oneness, permit itself to be perceived by us as having parts?

RH: Illusion! Does Oneness come to you and say, "Hey! Look at my parts"? No. *You* are dreaming about non-existent "parts."

There is no division, no modification, no multiplicity, no diversity. That there appear to be such things as "parts" is the grand illusion, what I call the "benign conspiracy." On a minute-to-minute basis, this conspiracy is reinforced by your fellow conspirators. They speak about the world and the things in it as "real," and their ordinary minds treat these things in a concrete manner. With each breath, distinctions and diversity are noted, emphasized, and encouraged. The

Oneness is forgotten, the not-self is promoted and worshiped. But as a seeker, you must withdraw from this conspiracy. You must turn inward and find out from *where* the distinctions emanate. Then you will Know that no divisions or distinctions are possible.

Student: It will become very difficult to continue with one's everyday life.

RH: A speculation of ordinary mind! Being ignorant of who you are and the nature of the world, as you admittedly are now, do you say you have trouble living your everyday life? No. How much better will you be able to live as one who abides in Self.

Student: But we will be so aware of the ignorance of others and of the nonsense we see all around us.

RH: More fantasies and diversions! Now your ordinary mind is depicting an illusory enlightened state for you. The only "nonsense" is that you have forgotten your true nature. Find out if there are "others" who are "ignorant." Abide as Self; then you can determine if you must change your life and turn away from the world.

RH: Let me show you something appropriate here.

(In response to Mr. Hittleman's request, an assistant hung on the wall the illustration that is reproduced on page 79.

This is a geometrical design known as a *yantra*. Fix your attention on it.

(There was a pause while the group studied the illustration.)

Who sees the white planes as the *tops* of the cubes?

(A number of students raised their hands.)

And who sees the white planes as the *bottoms* of the cubes?

(Others raised their hands.)

Now, can you exchange your view? That is, can those of you who are seeing the white planes as the tops of the cubes see them as the bottoms, and vice versa?

(There was a pause and some discussion among

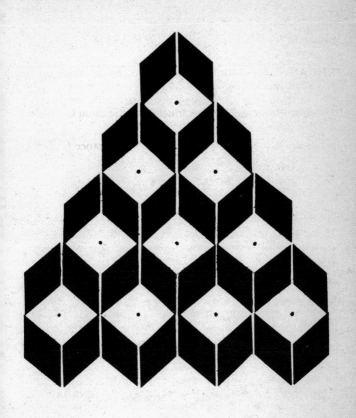

YANTRA

the students, but it appears that all were able to make the exchange in their perception. Most of the group were then able to go back and forth between the two perceptions.)

So, you see how it is: nothing in the yantra changes; only your *perception* changes. While it is inaccurate to say that "Self perceives," this yantra demonstrates how the instantaneous change of perception occurs. You don't "make progress" toward this change. It happens *suddenly*.

Now, tell me this: can anyone see the white planes as both the tops and the bottoms of the cubes simultaneously?

(After an interval of observation and discussion, it was agreed that none were able to have this simultaneous perception.)

So, although your perception changes *instantaneously*, that is, although you may see the white planes as the tops of the cubes, and the very next second see them as the bottoms, you cannot see them simultaneously. In the same way, you cannot see the world as the world—that is, in multiplicity and diversity—and simultaneously abide as Self.

RH: Earlier today, someone told me that she was attending this workshop because she recently had a realization that she was not getting what she wanted out of life. I thought this expression, "getting what I want out of life," was worth commenting upon because we hear it so often. It is a popular statement of the conspirators.

The gist is this: life is depicted as an entity somewhat like a giant department store brimming with innumerable products. You wade into this container of indispensable goodies and, according to your pocketbook, "get" or "not get" what you want out of it. But the Truth is that life is not apart from the one who lives. Existence manifests spontaneously each moment and there is only the experience of existing, not of existing "in a life." An understanding of this will be extremely significant to the student because it aids in quieting the mind and turning it inward. You see, if

---

one believes that life is something external or apart from existence, that is, something that can be grasped and manipulated, then all one's efforts are directed toward fulfilling desires in an illusory world. You cannot "get" anything out of life and you cannot "give" anything to life. You cannot live a "full" life and you cannot live an "empty" life. You can only BE. An understanding that you ARE maintains your ONENESS. But believing that you *are this or that*, or that you *can become this or that*, engenders the desire to manifest as something other than what you ARE. Any such effort is futile. You can only BE.

Another Student: That is certainly contrary to the way in which just about everybody thinks. Probably half the world is involved in self-improvement of some kind.

RH: First see if you have a "self." Then you will know if it requires "improvement."

Student: I mean that almost everyone wants to function more effectively in one way or another.

RH: Yes. A fundamental proposition of the conspiracy is that "self-improvement" results in increased satisfaction and that it may even result in fulfillment. So do what you must do. But be aware that no action or thought can alter your BEING. Whether you believe that you are functioning effectively or ineffectively, you are always Self. Abide as Self and you will know peace.

Another Student: Are you saying that we shouldn't attempt to do anything along self-improvement lines?

RH: "Self-improvement" is a cherished concept of the conspiracy because there is no end to it. The ordinary mind can keep you effectively preoccupied with self-improvement for a multitude of lifetimes. People often become indignant when I speak of self-improvement as a "futile effort." Do whatever you must do, but reflect for a moment on this: Who will do the "improving" of the "self"?

Student: I will.

RH: So you mean that there is an "I" who is going to "improve" a "self"? That means there are two selves: one that needs improving and another that is going to do the improving. Correct?

(The student did not reply.)

RH: Now tell me this: who will decide whether or not the "improving" process is proceeding satisfactorily?

Student: I will.

RH: Is that the "I" who needs to be improved or is that the I who is going to do the improving? If it is neither, then there must be three selves: one who needs to be improved, one who will do the improving, and one who will act as the observer to see if the improving is proceeding properly.

(Laughter)

And who will sit in judgment on the third "I" to determine if he is making the correct evaluation as to whether the improvement is satisfactory?

(The student did not reply.)

RH: So you see, there are no end to these selves. You have divided Self into all of these selves and you no longer know who you are. Self requires no improving; it could never be other than Whole and Perfect.

Another Student: I would think that this knowledge would make you want to withdraw from the world.

RH: Well, you have the knowledge now. Are you ready to withdraw from the world?

Student: No, but I don't really have the knowledge; I mean, the experience.

RH: Exactly. The "knowledge" means very little, although it may help. But the *experience* is the thing. So *experience* Self. Experience Self by BEING Self. Then the question of whether or not to withdraw will no longer arise.

Student: Why not?

RH: The ordinary mind conceives "withdrawal" as "abandonment," as "pulling out." But Self does not enter and it does not exit. You ARE Self and, as such, there is no possibility of involvement or withdrawal.

Student: If a significant number of people were unconcerned as to whether or not they were functioning efficiently, wouldn't there be a real deterioration of the society?

RH: Do you see such indifference now manifesting in the society as the result of our teachings?

Student: No, but probably only a relatively very small number are exposed to this philosophy.

RH: Well, that's comforting. Have no fear. I won't tell if you don't.
(Laughter)
Understand first *who* is concerned with deterioration and you will have an insight into the fear tactics of ordinary mind.

Student: Are *you* [meaning RH] an illusion of my ordinary mind?

RH: Everything that proceeds from ordinary mind is transient and, therefore, unreal; being unreal, it is an illusion.

Student: You mean that as I am seeing you now, you are an illusion, and if I see you from Self you are real?

RH: These questions can be the product only of ordinary mind. Your questioning my reality is based on the ordinary mind's assumption that we are separate. As Self there is only ONENESS without separation, without division. As Self, you cannot "see" me either as "real" or as an "illusion." There is no Self-objectification, that is, there is no subject to "see" an object. All is Self.

Another Student: When you are absorbed in Self, do you maintain any sense of individuality?

RH: At no time do you have any "individuality" to main-

---

tain. "Individuality" is synonymous with "self." You must not be afraid of losing what you do not have.

Student: It seems to me that a great deal of practice is necessary to make the mind sufficiently subtle to be receptive to this philosophy.

RH (After a pause): Excuse me a moment.

(Mr. Hittleman stood up and walked to a nearby table. He took an orange from a bowl of fruit and returned to his place. He resumed a seated position and began to examine the orange.)

No. You need not be concerned with the receptivity of your mind.

(The student to whom he was speaking was seated approximately ten feet from him. Without warning, Mr. Hittleman tossed the orange at the student. It was an easy toss; the orange was meant to be caught, and it was. The student was startled and everyone laughed.)

Good catch! How did you do it? Did you analyze the trajectory?

Student (Smiling): No.

RH: Did you compute the wind interference?

(The student shook his head no, still smiling.)

RH: So, you made no preparations. Your present "situation" in life was totally forgotten. You saw the orange coming, you put out your hands, and you caught it. In the same way, you need not prepare your mind; it doesn't have to be made "subtle" or "receptive." Self is coming toward you at each moment. Put out your hands and "catch" it.

Another Student: This may be stretching the point, but actually he *did* make various mental preparations to catch the orange. It's just that they occurred so rapidly that you don't realize all that was involved.

RH: Yes, just as you don't realize that *you* have already made all the necessary preparations to BE. Nothing more need be done.

The Student who caught the orange: What if I hadn't caught it?

RH: There was no such possibility.

Student: How is that?

RH: Remain in the center and you will comprehend that there are no "possibilities." There is only what IS.

Another Student: But there are an infinite number of choices that one can make. How can you say, "There are no possibilities"?

RH: "Possibilities" are the property of the computer, the ordinary mind. As such, they are indeed infinite. But You ARE. In Reality, you act—or what the ordinary mind construes as "action"—from the center, as Self, not according to "possibilities." Recognize omnipresent ONENESS and you will not be sucked into the illusion by "possibilities." No matter what you do, it is the only thing you *can* do. If, in the course of BEING, you suddenly allow the illusion of "possibilities" to convince you that you might do or be other than you ARE, your ONENESS is obscured.

You have come to worship your ordinary mind precisely because it *can* present you with these infinite possibilities. "How wonderful," you say. You fail to recognize that the illusion of these possibilities does not foster freedom but actually holds you in bondage.

Student: I cannot choose?

RH: Why burden yourself with the illusion of choices? Throughout an infinite number of lifetimes the ordinary mind will torment you not only with "possibilities" and "choices," but with the concern as to whether you have made the *right* choice. And what is it that evaluates the right or wrong of a choice?—*the very instrument that is presenting the endless choices:* ordinary mind. These "possibilities," which you find so desirable and important, are creations of the ordinary mind. Why worship them and perpetuate your enslavement? Know that, mercifully, you cannot be *this or that*; you can only BE. In Truth, whatever you *appear* to do is proceeding from your ONENESS, not from the illusion that you have made a choice among possibilities.

Another Student: I believe I'm not alone in my experience of having acted in a particular manner and being displeased with the results. I think about it and decide that next time, in a similar situation, I'll act differently. I *do* act differently and the outcome is much more satisfactory. I consciously *chose* to act differently.

RH: Why all this ordinary-mind analysis of "right" and "wrong"? Why do some people regard a thing as "right" and others regard the same thing as "wrong"? And why do people regard the same thing as "right" at one time and "wrong" at another? If something is True, Right, would not everyone always regard it as so? Abandon these games of the computer. Remain in your ONENESS as Self and you will no longer be subject to the tyranny of the ordinary mind's "right" and "wrong." If you are unable to recognize the Truth of your ONENESS, NOW, then at least find out *who* is this "I" that you speak of as "choosing" and "acting."

Student: Why does God permit war, famine, and suffering?

RH: Why ask me? Ask Him.

Student (After a pause): I don't know how.

RH: But you say that you know He permits war, famine, and suffering?

(The student did not reply.)

RH: Does war come to you and say, "God has permitted me to manifest"?

Student: If God is all, then such things must exist with His sanction.

RH: Find out if they "exist" before you bother God about them. If you are unable to *ask* Him a simple question such as why He permits war, famine, and suffering, then you had better satisfy your curiosity through other means.

Student: How?

RH: *Who* asks the question about war and suffering?

Student: *I* do.

RH: Turn the ordinary mind inward and trace this "I" that you speak of to its source. At the place where the I arises you will be able to ask your question—if you still find it necessary to do so.

Student: I want you and everyone in this room to know how much being here has meant to me. Your literature about this workshop came to me just at a time when it is necessary for me to make a major change in my life. Being here has helped me to see my situation in a completely different light. I really feel that my coming here was meant to be.

RH: Well, I'm pleased that these meetings have been helpful to you.

We have already spoken about "changes" and "decisions" and I trust you'll recall what was said. But I would like to comment on your phrase "it was meant to be." It's another expression that we frequently hear and we should take a moment to examine it.

If you lend credence to the idea that "it was meant to be," then you obviously believe that there are innumerable situations and occurrences which were *not* meant to be. This reinforces the ordinary mind's illusion of "destiny"; it emphasizes that existence is fraught with chance, that it is the product of an entity which creates man and disinterestedly watches him "sink or swim." Sometimes man's "luck" is good and the dice roll well for him. At other times, he stumbles about, subject to the whims of "fortune," desperately attempting to "master his fate," informed on all sides by the conspirators that he is only a "speck in the universe," and so forth. All these words and phrases effectively keep him a slave of the ordinary mind because it is able to convince him, again and again, that he is obviously in need of continual assistance in order to navigate through this maze of "chance." The ordinary mind nominates itself as the entity which will provide such guidance; it seconds its own nomination and elects itself unanimously.

When certain circumstances are analyzed by the ordinary mind in a particular way, something "clicks" and you interpret this experience as one that "was *meant* to be." By *whom* was it "meant to be"? Has some entity arranged these particular events so that they become "meaningful" to it? If this is the case, are all other occurrences *less* meaningful or *not* meaningful to it? The Truth is that there is nothing that was *meant* to be, and nothing that was *not* meant to be, and nothing that was *meant to be more* than something else. ALL simply IS. As long as you fail to BE-ALL-NOW, you will imagine yourself a "pawn in the game," waiting for your "ship to come in," looking to get a "break," wondering, "Why did this happen to me?" and, as a "speck in the universe," vulnerable to everything that can "go wrong." So, remain as Self and no such illusions can arise.

Student: Is Self attained only while one is living in the body or can it be attained from the other states as well?

RH: Remember that you are *always* Self and that there is nothing to "attain." Since Self IS all that you have ever sought, or are now seeking, or *will* seek in the illusory past-present-future sequence, why not recognize Self NOW? Why concern yourself with different "states" of existence?

(Pause)

However, to accommodate your ordinary mind, let me add that many of the Eastern scriptures inform us that enlightenment can manifest only while one is incarnate. They also observe that an incarnation is a rare thing, not easily come by. All this is to emphasize the urgency of devoting one's most serious efforts to the business of Self-recognition in *this* lifetime.

Student: If one achieves the enlightened state during her lifetime, does she continue to live? I mean, "live" in the usual sense of the word.

RH: She continues to act as the manifestation of her previous karma requires her to act. Unless she actually functions as a teacher, she will appear no different from the ordinary person and no different from the person she was prior to this "enlightenment." Only *another* enlightened being recognizes her. A person who is Self-recognized and who, therefore, functions as Universal Mind, generates no new karma while her previous karma is dissipating. But, understand that an enlightened person no longer sees herself as confined to a body, and she is totally unconcerned with the concept of karma. The ordinary person feels that she is encompassed within a body, and so she believes that one who is enlightened [*jnani*] must also be in a body. That is the point of view from which you asked the question. One who has failed to recognize her true nature cannot Know the state of the *jnani*.

Another Student: If a person *does* proclaim the fact of his enlightenment and becomes a teacher or a guru, how are we to believe that his enlightenment and teachings are genuine?

RH: If a person announces, "I am enlightened," or, "I am a guru," it is usually best to leave his presence as quickly as possible. In other words, "Run for it."
  (Laughter)
  One who is abiding in Self does not consider himself "enlightened" or apart from others. As far as your knowing if his or her teachings are genuine, trust your intuition. You will intuitively know if this instruction is emanating from the center and you will feel it if his presence imparts the quietude you are seeking. This instruction [*darshan*] may be verbal or silent or both. You may perceive these things instantaneously or you may require some period of exposure to him. But ultimately, you will know.

Another Student: I know that *you* are a guru.

RH: In the same way you are. Each person is both the student and the guru of the next.

Student: You have been my guru for many years, through your books and recordings.

(Mr. Hittleman nodded but did not reply.)

Another Student: Listen, Richard. I know that most people here won't say this—even though they may think it—and I understand why *you* won't say it, but let's face it: there sure are a lot of phonies and fakers around. That bizarre appearance of that boy guru in the Astrodome, and the bands of kids roaming through the streets with shaven heads, distributing pamphlets and proselytizing, and those Hindus who come from India and spend a week or two in someone's home and set it up as a "center" and then go on to the next city and establish the next "center" and solicit donations to send back to India . . .you know, I've been around for a long time and I wouldn't give you a dime for ninety-nine percent of the so-called gurus, Hindu or otherwise. I don't want to offend anyone here, but I'm telling it like I see it.

RH: Well, I'm sure most of us understand what you wish to convey, but we must have the correct perspective of these things. The world of the ordinary mind is no different from the way it has always been and always will be. There are those who are seeking, and so teachers and sects manifest on what appears to be many different levels of understanding to meet the needs of the various seekers. It is true that young people of high-school and college age may tend to be more gullible and indiscriminate in their spiritual quest, and this is true simply because they *are* young and lack experience. But many will gain the necessary experience to understand the pure doctrine by doing exactly what they *are* doing.

Young people tend to be attracted by certain "trappings." They are drawn to chanting, robes, sandals, incense, dark rooms, colored lights, music, parades,

Hindus, Caucasians who have taken or been given Hindu names, and so forth. Some of these young people are in reaction to their environment, some are looking for a "far-out blast" that simulates a drug experience, and some are simply following their peers and doing the "in" thing; but many are intensely serious and dedicated. *All* who say they are "seeking" must always be given the benefit of any doubt you may have. Understand that everything is always exactly as it must be. If you don't recognize this truth, you will believe that "chance" and "error" are realities and you will become preoccupied with why and how the society should be "improved."

When I have occasion to tell a group of young people that the robes, sandals, incense, and so forth are unnecessary and can even be obstacles to their practice, I note that many of the group are disappointed. It's as if I've eliminated much of the romance and adventure of the quest. They lack the experience to discern *where* the true adventure lies. Also, I note that many of these groups of young people are uncertain as to how they should evaluate me. I come before them just as you see me now, with relatively short hair, beardless, in Western clothes, without a Hindu name. I usually speak while seated at a table—not on the floor—without flowers, beads, or incense. This is simply my way. I have not found it necessary to adopt these various "trappings," although there is certainly nothing wrong with them, providing you do not begin to mistake the trappings for the doctrine.

Another Student: I make use of incense and flowers in the room I use for my Yoga practice and meditation. They create very pleasant, relaxing vibrations.

RH: Yes, that's perfectly acceptable, and especially so if you find that these "vibrations" assist in the quieting of your mind. Be aware, however, that it's your mind that creates the vibrations, not the flowers. All external trappings that aid in creating an atmosphere in which the mind can be stilled are acceptable. But one must understand that having a pleasant, relaxed feeling is not the meditation of our doctrine. Turning the mind inward and determining its source is the practice. Once you become seriously involved in this, the external setting of your practice will be of no consequence and a coal cellar will be the same as a temple.

Another Student: Do you have disciples?

RH: I don't encourage this disciple-teacher relationship in the classical sense. There are those who do; it is simply not my way. I meet with people, like yourselves, from time to time and tell them what I am telling you. I urge them to turn inward and to discover that they are their *own* gurus. I present the various techniques, such as those of the Yogas, that may be helpful in this regard.

Student: Do you have—or did you have—a guru?

RH: All who pushed me from outside and forced me to turn inward have been my gurus.

Student: I mean, was there a particular guru?

RH: I know what you mean. . . . Ramana Maharshi.

Student: Can you tell us some of your experiences?

RH: No. It is not my way to speak of these things. There are those who do recount experiences with their gurus.

Another Student: I think you should have a permanent center where you might be accessible to those who, like myself, want to see you more often than once or twice a year.

RH: It has been my experience that the various Yoga centers, *ashrams,* retreats, and so forth that have been established in this country have not proven satisfactory for conveying the ultimate and unadulterated doctrine of Self-recognition.

Student: Why is this?

RH: Essentially, it has to do with what is involved in the process of organizing and maintaining these institutions. At every point the institution must reflect the spirit of the master around whom it has been organized. This requires great skill and knowledge.

Those who are charged with the responsibility of organizing and maintaining must be so utterly imbued with the spirit of the master that his teachings pervade everything: the kitchen, the business office, the social events, and the multitude of other aspects. However, it has been my observation that such is not the case and that these "centers" either fall apart from lack of this spirit, or congeal in a way that requires them to assume all the dynamics of the corporate structure: grievances, petty differences, struggles for power, and desire for favor and recognition are frequently prevalent. Also, for many, the ashram functions as a "crutch" and can become as much of an obstruction as an aid in Self-recognition. What I have just stated is a generalization derived from my own observations. Of course, there may be exceptions.

Student: Are there gurus who have no ashrams?

RH: Gurus present their teachings in many situations. Some are wanderers and teach where and how they will. Jesus was such a guru. Some arrange a schedule of appearances at one or more places. Some have one or more ashrams and travel among them. Some have ashrams and remain there permanently. Then, there are those who instruct and guide without any personal contact with students. This is all a matter of the style of the particular guru.

Student: What do you think of going to India? Do you advise it?

RH: These things are contingent on one's attraction. If you are being irresistibly drawn there, then go. Otherwise, stay home quietly and BE.

Student: Is there a particular ashram you could recommend?

RH: I recommend the ashram you find when you turn inward, when you "go into your closet." If you feel that you require a special external environment in order to become internalized, then you must seek one. But, whether you go or stay, you are always Self.

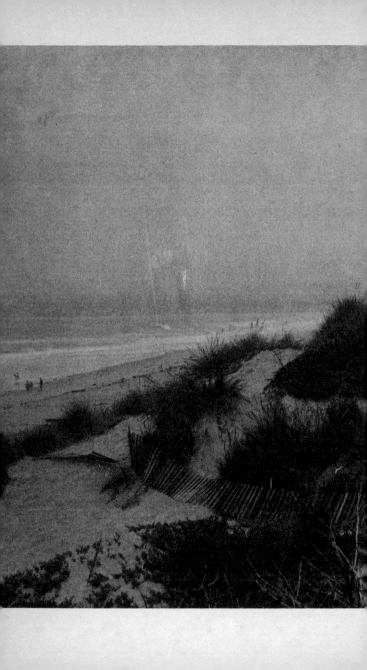

4th day

Student: As you know, I teach *Comparative Philosophy*. Much of what you are presenting here is *advaita* [non-duality]. This can be classified as the philosophy of Vedanta. You are also instructing us in the Yoga techniques. Yoga postulates the principle of self [duality] that must merge with Self. Therefore, Yoga and Vedanta are considered two different schools. Do you reconcile the differences in these two schools to the student?

RH: All such illusory "differences" are reconciled in *practice*. "Schools" and "classifications" are for scholars. Those who function in the center teach what they *experience*, what they Know Absolutely. Scholars examine, interpret, and classify these teachings and structure "schools" around them. But Self-recognition does not transpire through a school; it is *direct* and *absolute*

Knowledge. Self makes no distinction among "schools." In truth, each teacher can be said to be a "school." He presents those techniques which have proven fruitful for him. He is unconcerned as to whether these techniques have been incorporated into "schools," just as he is unconcerned as to whether scholars have judged these schools as having "different points of view." The student may accept or reject the instruction of the teacher, but it would be the greatest folly to do either on the basis of whether the teacher conformed to the principles of a particular "school." The distinctions that are noted by academicians are superficial. Both philosophies are primarily concerned with eliminating the unreal, the not-Self. The "duality" of Yoga and the "nonduality" of Vedanta are concepts for the accommodation of ordinary mind. For Self, there are no such concepts. All the *shastras*, the *Vedas* and *Upanishads* as well as the epics such as the *Mahabharata*, from which the *Bhagavad-Gita* is an excerpt, proceed from the ONE. The teacher, to accommodate the ordinary mind of the student, may speak of the wisdom contained in these scriptures as various "points of view" or varying "approaches." But all are of Self.

Another Student: You use a number of different terms for "Self." Are these all synonyms or does each have a different shade of meaning?

RH: They can all be considered identical. Self has no "shades." There are various words and phrases utilized in different texts and sects to indicate Self. I speak to people who, because of their previous studies and practices, have varying points of reference. So I employ these different words for their convenience. Universal Mind, Pure Consciousness, Unconditioned Intelligence, God, Brahma, Buddha, Oneness, Absolute—all are Self.

In addition, there are words and phrases that I use as synonyms to indicate the temporal process of *self having fused with Self:* Self-consciousness, Self-recognition, Self-awareness, absorption, Yoga, samadhi, satori, quietude, peace, integration, center of the circle, mergence, bliss, nirvana, enlightenment, and others that I don't recall just now.

Student: Isn't *nirvana* a Buddhist word?

RH: It is a Sanskrit term, which, although found in numerous Hindu scriptures [including the Hatha Yoga texts and the *Bhagavad-Gita*], is employed by Buddhists to represent the ultimate objective. It means "blown out," and the imagery is that of a fire which is extinguished when there is no longer fuel upon which it can feed. The "fire" is the way in which the ordinary man acts and suffers in maya. The "fuel" consists of the illusions generated by ordinary mind. Therefore, the fire (suffering) is extinguished when the fuel (ordinary mind) is no longer supplied. In this connection it is important to note Patanjali actually defines the whole of Yoga as "the restraining of the changes [movements] of mind." Can you grasp the profound simplicity of this? It means, quiet your mind and keep it quiet and there is Yoga!

Student: Is there such a thing as a "conscience"? I mean, is conscience actually Self that attempts to advise us?

RH: No. Conscience is not the nature of Self. What you think of as your "conscience" is ordinary mind playing with ordinary mind.

Student: But it seems that there is *something* that is able to point out the right path when we take—or think about taking—the wrong one. Frequently, we are about to do something that is to our disadvantage and a voice tells us to stop and reconsider.

RH: That is all the play of the ordinary mind. The so-called conscience is just another "I." You say, "My conscience tells me . . ." Which is the *real* I—the one who is advising or the one who is being advised?

Student (After a pause): They're both me.

RH: So you are really talking to yourself. Find out *who* the "self" is that you are talking to and you will no longer be troubled by "right path" and "wrong path."

Student: What would you say are the ideal conditions for undertaking the practice of Yoga very seriously?

RH: If you seek the "ideal conditions" you will neglect your practice. There is no moment at which you are unable to turn the mind inward. Therefore, *all* conditions are "ideal."

Student: There are certain conditions that are obviously preferable: minimal external distractions such as noise and so forth, and a minimum of obligations, and minimal concern about money, health, and so forth.

RH: All these things you mention are conjurings of the ordinary mind to forestall your practice. The longer it can put you off with "certain conditions," the less threatened is its position. It has been my experience that those who seek "ideal conditions" never find them. They are always "just on the verge" of becoming serious, but months and years pass and they remain "just on the verge." It is the ordinary mind which seeks "ideal conditions." Self is *un-conditioned*. Self is HERE, NOW.

Student: Being here this week and having access to the Hatha Yoga classes, to meetings with you, to the special meals, to the beach and ocean, and being among others who have the same objectives as myself, have made a big difference. I feel that I've made much more progress than I do at home. I know you don't approve of the word *progress* but I don't know how else to express it.

RH: The situation that you find here this week is a contrived one. It is the purposeful arrangement of certain elements that become a format for conveying particular knowledge in a particular way. But this knowledge fulfills its purpose only when it is applied in your ordinary, everyday life, not in a perpetually contrived situation.

So now you have the necessary knowledge. It is also available from my books and recordings, and those of others. Go home and apply what you know to your everyday life.

Student: My life at home is complicated. I have many family obligations. I cannot always find the time to practice as I should. Also, I do not have a separate room where I can practice quietly. It's very frustrating. I've even thought about running away from home for a while.

(Many members of the group expressed their agreement with these statements. Several described similar situations.)

RH: If you should run away from home and travel to the Himalaya Mountains and crawl into a cave—there you will come face to face with your obligations. Wherever you run, the ordinary mind runs with you. You must do what has come to you to do, at home, at your place of work, or wherever else, to the best of your ability. All your work should become "active meditation." The ordinary mind may be turned inward and fixed there, wherever you are. Why waste your time bemoaning your karma? If you think you have "complications" and "obstacles," then you must make all the more effort.

It is a natural law, more certain than that of gravity, that one who undertakes to practice seriously, no matter what his or her circumstances, soon finds that these circumstances are altered so that practice can be accommodated. Make it a point to practice whenever you can; practice in five-minute segments if necessary. The same forces that are responsible for what you now interpret as "complications" and "obligations" will arrange circumstances to accommodate your practice requirements. Of this there is not the slightest doubt.

Another Student: Many sages advise students to simplify their lives, to divest themselves of possessions and obligations.

RH: Such divesting may have a certain romantic appeal to the novice, but, in reality, the ordinary mind cannot simplify. Simplification results from turning the ordinary mind inward and fixing it there. Whenever you do this, you will find that there are no complications. Your possessions are of no consequence; the manner in which you *regard* these possessions is everything. If you are attached to these possessions and objectify them as *belonging* to you, then they enslave you. You are buried in materialism. "Simplification," therefore, does not result from the physical act of relinquishing possessions and abandoning obligations, but from renunciation of the ordinary mind. In effect, it is renounced when it is turned inward.

Another Student: I'm a salesman. I'm on the road about four days each week and I must make a certain number of sales. When I'm talking to a customer and discussing an order with him, how can I turn my mind inward and quiet it? How could I do my work?

RH: The ordinary mind has convinced you that it is indispensable in your activities. You are assuming that *you* do the work and that the ordinary mind tells you *how* to do it. But through your practice you will come to recognize that neither is the case. You are Self and *Self does not act.* Your business with your customers will transpire as it must without your concern as to whether or not your "mind" is functioning. An inward-turned, quieted mind does not imply an inert and incompetent existence.

Student: I seem to require an incentive or a "push" in order to practice regularly—not always, but from time to time. I mean, there are days when I just don't seem able to bring myself to do it.

RH: Do what you can, whenever you can. All will be well. Whenever you require a "push," just consider the situation in which you find yourself: subject to the interminable cycle of birth and death; suffering throughout each incarnation; experiencing continual insecurity, frustration, and unrest. Once you begin to perceive the nature of the ordinary mind and of your existence in maya, you will have all the "push" that is necessary.

Another Student: In order to practice with the seriousness and dedication you advise, must we not have the *desire* to do so? If so, is this type of desire different from the "desire" we discussed previously?

RH: Remain as Self and there is no desire; all is already fulfilled. If you are unable to recognize this, then channel all your desires into *one* desire: the desire for Self-awareness. Hold this desire above all other desires and the others will subside. Ultimately, this one remaining desire will be consumed in Self.

Another Student: What about personality problems as they relate to Yoga practice? I know I have a problem with my temper. I've learned to control it pretty well, but I still become angry with others and especially with myself. If I'm unable to do a posture correctly on a particular day, or if my mind keeps distracting me in meditation, I become angry and frustrated, and I'm unable to continue. Do you have any suggestions?

RH: The emotions are precipitated by the ordinary mind. When you turn the mind inward, the emotions are also quieted. Each time the mind is turned inward for active or passive meditation, it is illuminated. Then, when it resumes its outward flow, it is less turbulent. In this way, the emotions become progressively tranquil and have diminishing power to disturb.

Student: Why should the mind resume its outward flow?

RH: It may not. One should always assume that it will not. Its tendency [*vasana*] to do so will be weakened each time you practice. At first, the mind seems to "jump" between inward and outward, but with continued practice your perception and sensitivity are refined to the point where you can actually detect the mind pulling to resume its outward flow. With such advance notice, your ability to prevent its outward flow greatly increases.

Another Student: When you say, "The emotions are tranquilized," do you mean *all* emotions?

RH: Yes.

Student: Happiness and joy as well? These are pleasurable emotions. Why should we want these to cease?

RH: What you are now thinking of as "happiness" is the opposite of "sorrow." The ordinary person's happiness is inherent in sorrow, and vice versa. She judges her happiness by the extent of the sorrow she has known, and vice versa. The emotional cycle of the ordinary mind is continuous, and, as the wheel turns, she experiences various degrees of emotional opposites. When she experiences what for her is the zenith of happiness, it is only a question of time until the turning wheel decreases this happiness and brings her into the realm of sorrow—perhaps to the depths of sorrow.
(Pause)
Do you know permanent happiness?

Student: No.

RH: But you seek it. And although all that you do is undertaken with this objective—to know permanent happiness and avoid pain and suffering—you have been unsuccessful. How do you account for this?

Student: Well, I know from listening to you that I've been looking in the wrong direction.

RH: Yes. The ordinary person seeks happiness in an external world that is created by her ordinary mind. Not perceiving that ordinary mind is an entity of endless change, she is unable to grasp the fact that varying degrees of happiness and tranquillity will perpetually alternate with varying degrees of sorrow and agitation. So, she experiences no lasting peace.

Your true nature is happiness—not the happiness which is the opposite of sorrow, but ultimate and permanent happiness. This happiness is better designated "bliss." Of course, you really do know—or at least strongly suspect—that bliss *is* your true nature, and that's why all your efforts are directed toward abiding in it. When you seek happiness in the conditions of the world, you are *really* seeking reintegration with this inner state of Unconditioned Bliss.

Searching for happiness in the conditions of the world is an utterly futile endeavor. The ordinary mind convinces you, again and again, that you haven't found this happiness because you haven't performed the right actions, acquired sufficient possessions, known the right people, secured the right employment, and so on, ad infinitum. You are held a prisoner in the world as you vainly seek happiness through the endless "possibilities" dredged up by ordinary mind. Therefore, relinquish these notions of "joy" and "happiness"; turn *inward* and you will Know the eternal Bliss of Self.

Another Student: Then we should attempt to attain emotional *balance*?

RH: The ancients taught, "Neither rejoice in your good fortune nor despair in your travail." They are advising the seeker to maintain emotional *quiescence*, to minimize his "ups" and "downs" by regarding what befalls him with *dispassion*—as the natural karmic law of cause and effect. The ordinary mind may tend to interpret this dispassionate view as detracting from the "joy" or "fun" of living. But even what the ordinary mind envisions as the wildest joy is short-lived and is soon transformed into sorrow. The greatest happiness that one derives from the conditions of the world is but the palest reflection of the sublime Bliss of Self. Therefore, turn the ordinary mind inward, quiet the emotions; abide as Self, and Bliss is Known.

Student: Doesn't Hatha Yoga help quiet the emotions?

RH: Very much so; especially the pranayama [breathing] techniques. Although pranayama is a temporary expedient, it assists in pointing the way.

Another Student: I'd like to pursue the "emotional" thing a little further. There are psychotherapists who advise us to "get in touch with our *real* feelings." How would this relate to what you were just saying?

RH: The imagery suggested by the statement is that of a layer of superficial feelings, underneath which lies the layer of "real" feelings. But the truth is that all emotions are associated with ordinary mind and none are more "real" than others. Wasn't it Oscar Levant who, in commenting on Hollywood, said, "Underneath all that phony tinsel is the *real* tinsel"? Everything that is of the not-Self is illusory. Everything of Self is Real. One who is mentally or emotionally ill may be helped by such "getting in touch" thereapy. But a search for one's "real" feelings will not result in Self-recognition.

Another Student: Am I correct in concluding from what you have said that we needn't concern ourselves with eliminating what are usually considered harmful or destructive personality traits?

RH: Concern yourself with whatever you will, but while you are involved in these things, don't forget to turn inward—to practice.

Student: You mean meditate.

RH: Yes, actively and passively. But also be aware that *dhyana* [meditation] is your true nature. You are always meditating. In the unenlightened state, from the circumference of the circle, it appears that one must practice meditation, practice Yoga. But once Self is recognized, that which was previously the means—the techniques—is suddenly transformed into the goal. When we say, "He is practicing Yoga," we mean that he is utilizing and applying the techniques of Yoga. But he is doing this so that he may *achieve* Yoga [reintegration]. At present, your ordinary mind conceives of "practicing meditation" as it thinks about any activity: in terms of time, place, and effort. But in *becoming* meditation, from the center of the circle, you understand that no effort has been necessary; you have always been meditating. *There is nothing you can do that is not meditation.*

Student: Are there degrees of enlightenment? Does the ordinary man pass through different *stages*?

RH: To the ordinary man, it *appears* so. The great synthe-
sizer of Yoga practices, Patanjali, actually describes
such stages of progression. I have discussed these
stages in my *8 Steps* book. *Stages*, *degrees*, and *progression* are words used to accommodate ordinary mind's
need for space and time input. In Reality, Self has no
degrees.

Another Student: Another question about "personality."
Should I not engage in any kind of self-analysis?

RH: You have no self. "Self-analysis" is like the magician
examining the illusion he has created. Do you need to
examine the garbage before you dispose of it? Where
will be the end to such self-analysis? Nonetheless,
analyze and examine whatever you need to, but be
aware that this is ordinary mind analyzing ordinary
mind. Your illusion of "self" is reinforced through
"self-analysis." The self will be dissolved only in your
recognition of Self.

Another Student: There are certain methods that are being
taught for "raising the consciousness." Are you famil-
iar with them?

RH: Your business is not to raise your consciousness but to
recognize your true nature. In the course of turning
inward, the consciousness will be transformed as
necessary. To deliberately undertake the raising of
consciousness—or any other similar practice—is to
lose sight of the true goal. *Who* will do the "raising"?
Are you two consciousnesses—one that needs to be
"raised" and one that will do the "raising"? Find out
who it is that wants to "raise the consciousness." When
you have found out *who*, you will no longer be concerned with the height of your consciousness.

Student: Isn't Kundalini Yoga a method to raise the consciousness?

RH: Kundalini Yoga prescribes certain practices through
which the kundalini *shakti* [force] is aroused and, in its
course of travel to unite with Siva [Yoga], is made to
pierce the six major *chakras* [centers]. In this process,

the consciousness is transformed, but this transformation is not the objective of the practice. Kundalini's mergence with Siva, which is Yoga, is the goal. The student is to view with *dispassion* whatever he finds transpiring in his consciousness during the Kundalini practice. *Who* is experiencing these phenomena?—*that* is the concern of the student.

Student: In some of your writings on *meditation*, you instruct the student to direct his consciousness to various things or places.

RH: Yes, always as an expedient, to give the ordinary mind something to fix upon so that it may become quiet, steady, and one-pointed.

Another Student: What is the difference between the "consciousness" and the "mind"?

RH: Consciousness is another word for "awareness." It can be considered as that through which we become *aware* of what is presented by mind.

Student: But my understanding, from what you have taught us, is that *there is only awareness*, and that mind is simply the *thought* of mind.

RH: Yes, an essential point. All these words are used for the purpose of giving mind something to grasp, to "attract" it so it cannot just dismiss these teachings as "totally incomprehensible" and, in this manner, evade exposure.

The ordinary mind functions in terms of space and time. Therefore, to accommodate the ordinary mind, we allow it to assume that thoughts arise from and are stored in *something*, and, further, that the information needed to function in and interpret the world is fed by the brain and senses into *something* where it is evaluated. This "something" we designate "mind." I refer to it as "ordinary mind" to indicate that it is a *limiting* entity.

So, for the ordinary man, the mind acts as a computer and the consciousness is the entity which becomes *aware* or *cognizant* of the computer's "readouts."

The word *subconsciousness* designates awareness on another level. Ordinary mind is responsible for creating the illusion of a "self," of multiple "I's," of an "ego," of Self being confined in a physical body—all of which appear to circumscribe Universal Mind and limit Awareness.

In our work we practice to turn the mind upon itself, to introvert it. As it turns inward we recognize that *we do not have a mind* in the usual sense of the word *mind*. All that we have, or rather, all that we *are*, is Unlimited and Infinite AWARENESS. Therefore, you are quite correct in saying that "there is only awareness"—if you understand what you are saying.

Another Student: What about the state that is designated "unconscious"?

RH: *Un* means "not." We can scarcely communicate about that which we believe *is*, so let us leave what "is not" alone.

Student: I mean, does the "I" exist in the unconscious state?

RH: The "I" does not exist, period. There is no "state" for it to exist *in*. ALL IS SELF. Whether awake, dreaming, or in deep sleep; whether conscious, sub-conscious, or unconscious you are only SELF.

Student: If you can't help disliking another person and you have to see him every day—I mean, he works in the same office—what's the best way to handle it? Should you try to learn to like him or should you just ignore him as much as you can?

RH: Have you been following our discussions here?

Student: This is the second time I've come in to these meetings. I was here on Monday.

RH: Well, turn the situation to your advantage. Ask yourself, "*Who* is it that doesn't like this man?" Not, "*Why* don't I like him?" or, "How can I *learn* to like him?" but, "*Who* is it that doesn't like him?" If you can find the an-

---

swer to this question your problem with him will be resolved.

Student: Just ask myself, "Who?"

RH: Don't just *ask* it, find the answer.

Student: I'm not sure I understand.

RH: Nothing could be easier. *Who* is the "I" who is "not sure" he understands? The thing which you believe to be the primary reality of your existence is "I." First, the "I" thought arises, and from this everything else proceeds. Rather than worry about your "problem" with this other man, determine *where* the problem originates. You will find that it arises at that place where the "I" arises. So find this place and you will discover that you have no problem at all!

Student: You mean that I'll see him differently, in a different way?

RH: You may not see him at all! Now you "see" everything, including the man you don't like, in a subject-object relationship. You say, "I'll (subject) see him (object)." Let us assume that the "I" who *sees* is no longer present. Then you cannot "see" anything, so you certainly can't see "him." If you no longer "see" him then surely your problem is resolved.

Student: What happens to him?

RH: Oh, so now you're worried about his welfare?
(Laughter)
Well, I'm not going to tell you what happens to him. I'm going to let you find out for yourself.

Student (Laughing): All right. I'll do my best. But he's going to be very surprised when he disappears!

RH (Laughing): So you'll have more revenge than you've hoped for!

Another Student: Then the crux of the matter is that if there is no more subject-object relationship, that other man ceases to be apart from Self.

RH: He was never apart from Self, no more than is our friend who has been asking the questions. In tracing the "I" to its source, you awaken from the dream of separation and diversity.

Student: For many years—this is when I was younger—I was obsessed with observing the teachings of Christ. It had to do in part with the way I was brought up and partly with my own genuine feelings of following in the footsteps of Christ. But it was a constant struggle and I was unhappy and filled with guilt. I was actually becoming ill. The church couldn't help me so I finally went to group therapy with a friend, and that helped me to realize that I could only be what I am and I shouldn't try to be something that I fantasized myself to be. Well, as I said, this was all quite some time ago, but since you speak about Jesus being a "Yogi," I'd like to hear your view of whether His teachings are really meant for everyone or are for just a very few people. How many people do you know who can truly "love his neighbor" or "turn the other cheek"?

RH: The Yogis speak of Jesus as a "Bhakta," meaning that He espoused the doctrine of love, humility, sacrifice, and surrender. But His teachings of this doctrine are for those with "ears to hear." For those who do not have such ears, this teaching is idealistic, impractical, naïve, impossible, and even masochistic. When the Bhakta turns the other cheek there is no question of "effort" involved. It is a manifestation of Self, of his being rooted in Self, of his acting from the center. Being Self, Jesus did not teach as one man speaking to other men and women. He spoke as Self, and those who have ears to hear are drawn into Self through the power of His words. What He is teaching you is that it is not a matter of judging that one has been "wronged" and making a deliberate decision to ignore this wrong-doing by "turning the other cheek." What the ordinary man may judge as "wrong," the Bhakta does not recognize as such, for judgment is not the nature of Self. Self dictates, "Judge not, that you be not judged."

Student: Then His teachings were *not* for all, but only for those who had "ears to hear"?

RH: All "hear" according to their levels of understanding. In your own case, His teachings precipitated an intense conflict, but this was all favorable because you eventually discovered that you could not take these teachings literally and turn the other cheek at will; you could not *impose* them on yourself. They must manifest as actions that flow from Self. Realizing this, you are now disposed to turning inward and seeking the *source* of the teachings.

Another Student: I don't mind saying that I absolutely can't stand people who fake being pious. I think that false piety is one of the most hypocritical, objectionable qualities there is. You see a lot of this "sweetness and light" sanctimonious pose among the Hindus and the young people who profess to be followers of the various gurus.

RH: The piety you are speaking of is *imposed*. Being imposed, it is recognized as unnatural and, therefore, "objectionable." Ironically, those whose self-image includes that of being a "pious" person frequently experience the greatest difficulty in turning inward.

Another Student: Why is that?

RH: Because those elements which comprise their "goodness" begin to dissolve before the illumination of Self and they have a difficult time in handling that. In other words, when the impostor is exposed to the Real, he realizes that his identity—or what he has considered his identity until now—can no longer be maintained. This fear of the loss of identity deters many from practicing seriously. The truth is, of course, that you have no identity to maintain. What you think of as your "identity" is a continually changing series of statistics fed to you by the computer, ordinary mind. When the mind is quieted, you are relieved of the oppressive burden of having to support an "identity."

Another Student: I've had the experience of loss of identity. I believe that Mrs. S—— mentioned the same thing the other day. It's the most fantastic experience, because you reach the point where you feel yourself, your identity, slipping away, and at that very moment you know that you've linked up with your *real* identity. It's as though your real identity is always there, but this other identity—your name and how you think about yourself and so forth—is covering it up.

Another Student (Questioning the one who had just spoken): And what happens then? How long do you remain as your *real* identity?

First Student: Well, It comes and goes. Once you've experienced it, you know it's always there, just as Mr. Hittleman was saying about the sun always shining. But it will seem to fade, and after a while return, and then fade again, and so forth. I'm speaking about what happens during my meditation. I have also had this experience when I'm doing my ordinary things, but not nearly as intensely. It occurs mostly during meditation.

RH: Continue your practice. It will manifest with increasing frequency.

Second Student (Continuing to question the first): And when this happens during your ordinary activities, can you continue to function as usual?

First Student: Oh, beautifully. It's like everything is absolutely perfect. Whatever work I'm doing seems to go on by itself.

Second Student: How long does it last?

First Student: A few minutes at a time. And then some days can go by and I won't have it, not even in meditation. But then it comes back, and when it's there it's as though it is *always* there. It's really difficult to explain.

Second Student: How long have you been meditating?

First Student: I've been practicing Hatha Yoga about two years and I've been meditating seriously about

. . . eight months. But I had this experience that I've just related to you during the first month I began the serious meditation.

RH: The element of "time" must never become a consideration in this work. In the beginning, you will be inclined to regard the practice as *leading* to an objective. Later, you will understand that *the practice is the objective.* Meditation is your true nature. Now, you are distinguishing between a time when you "meditate" and a time when you are engaged in your "ordinary things." As you continue to practice, this distinction will dissolve, and whether you are sitting quietly or doing what you must do in the world, you will know that *all is meditation.*

Student: I'm very interested in hearing more about the "loss of identity." Painting is my hobby—it's really more than a "hobby" because I'm extremely serious about it—and I remember that in one of your books you stated that the greatest works of art were executed by those who had lost their identity . . . it's probably better expressed as "transcended the self."

RH: Of course. Haven't you experienced that this is the case?

Student: I'm not sure. When I read your statements I attempted to contact the "center" as you described, and to execute my paintings from that center. But I'm not sure I succeeded. I would appreciate your giving me some additional information.

RH: You cannot "not be sure." When you are painting without an ego, from the center, as Self, there is no question as to whether or not you are doing so. The ego, the I, is an impediment in pure creation. As long as one believes "*I* am painting," the work that is produced will be imitative and uninspired. When your painting proceeds from the center, the I is no longer present. The work flows without the interference of ordinary mind. As such, it is Self-expression. Those creations which endure through the ages yet are

---

forever new and inspirational are Self-executed. At present, the Japanese are probably the most adept at executing art as a form of "active meditation." They also apply this principle to the martial arts.

Student: What is the technique for "centering"?

RH: "Self" and "center" are synonymous. Transcend the ego and you are in the center. You are *always* in the center as Self. We speak in terms of "center" and "circumference" to accommodate ordinary mind. We cater to it, but simultaneously we weaken its grasp.

Student: (After a pause): Were—and are—all great artists—those whom we call "genuises"—creating from Self?

RH: All are Self. All are always Self and nothing other.

Student: I don't know that as well as I would like to, especially when I'm painting.

RH: It is possible that these "genuises" of whom you speak labored under the same delusion. Their ordinary minds were transcended for certain intervals and then remanifested. They may not have recognized the permanence of the egoless condition, in the same way you are saying that you do not. But rather then speculate as to the state of others, you should attend fully to your own reality.

Another Student: If Self is ALL, how can there be art that is created apart from Self?

RH: The illusion that one has a "self" prevents him from creating in the egoless condition. All work that is performed with the sense of "*I* am working, *I* am creating" proceeds *without* Self-recognition.

Another Student: It seems to me that art would be the highest expression of Self.

RH: Self has no gradations. Ordinary mind must function in terms of "higher" and "lower." But when one abides in Self, *everything* is the "highest."

Another Student: So, all types of work and all jobs are of equal importance?

RH: Not "importance," just "equal." Find out *who* is doing the work and the question of its importance will not arise.

Student: I have several close friends who have changed their jobs because they felt that their previous jobs were incompatible with Yoga practice. Actually, I'm thinking of making a change myself.

RH: Let me remind you of certain very profound and subtle teachings of our doctrine: it is imperative that Yoga students become aware of the illusory nature of cause and effect so that they cease to reinforce them. *At all times, everything is precisely the only way it can BE.* To lend credence to the idea that things evolve or develop from other things, that circumstances and conditions have come about because of previous circumstances and conditions, and that these will evolve into future circumstances and conditions, is to reinforce the illusion of space and time, cause and effect, permanence and impermanence. Your changing of jobs is not the result of your Yoga practice or of anything else. If you change jobs it is because you change jobs. If you ascribe events to "causes" you perpetuate the ordinary mind's control; you are forever committed to attempt to arrange causes so that certain effects will manifest.

Those circumstances and qualities which now make something attractive and desirable, something worth the devotion of all your attention and labors, are changing. Because these circumstances cannot endure, the attraction cannot endure. Therefore, the ordinary man's *new* attractions—the need for new possessions, new situations, new activities—are interminable. These endless attractions and desires are the reasons for your bondage, suffering, and unrest.

Another Student: But karma *is* the doctrine of cause and effect. You have frequently alluded to karma in various explanations.

RH: Only as it is efficacious in aborting ordinary mind. Ordinary mind accepts the concept of karma exactly because it *is* comprised of the principle of cause and effect. Frequently, we can cut short what threatens to be a lengthy and unfruitful discussion of ordinary mind's curiosities by attributing something to "karma." This word satisfies ordinary mind and it may be temporarily stilled. We quiet it for a moment so that we may "push" it inward.

Student (After a pause): Yes, I see. This really is a subtle doctrine. The ordinary mind is tenacious; it pops up at every turn. As quickly as you believe you have transcended it, it's back with more questions . . . more doubts . . . more rationalizations. It surely doesn't want to be quiet.

RH: You can think of it as a group of legislators which is being pressured by the citizens it supposedly represents to pass a bill that will reduce its powers. You can understand that this legislative body will not be overly anxious to enact such legislation. Innumerable loopholes will be found to ensure delays and even a filibuster may be implemented. Similarly, when the ordinary mind perceives that its position of power and dominance is being threatened, it will squirm out of the threatening situation in any way it can.

Student: So, when you tell us that everything is always exactly as it must be, you're really saying that we should just let everything be as it is.

RH: Everything IS exactly as it IS regardless of whether or not you "let" it. You are not apart from that which IS. You ARE that which IS. Self is All.

Student: And we should make no effort to change anything?

RH: Find out *who* wants to make the changes. Then you will Know if the changes are necessary.

Another Student: You said before that "all work is equal."

Do you mean that a garbage collector's work is equal to that of a surgeon who saves someone's life by performing a highly skillful brain operation?

RH: A prevalent myth of the conspiracy is that there are gradations of importance in regard to work. The ordinary mind invents a value scale and proceeds to judge various situations or jobs as "noble, purposeful, exciting, important, indispensable," or "base, mundane, meaningless, unimportant, routine, boring." In short, ordinary mind would have one believe that there is work which is "desirable," and that there is work which is "undesirable." For most people, this belief sustains their restlessness and dissatisfaction. The garbage man and the brain surgeon are equally rooted in Self. The garbage man who does his work in the egoless condition, free from the fruits of his action, is, in the scriptures, viewed as superior to the brain surgeon who thinks, "What a marvelous operation *I* have performed." Ultimately, what a person does is inconsequential; how he *regards* what has befallen him to do is the index of his *understanding*.

Student: Is it wrong to want to be happy?

RH: Your original, true, pure, spotless, immutable nature is that of Happiness. You have no need to seek it. Discard all that is of the not-self and Happiness emerges. The "happiness" of which you are now speaking is the opposite of "unhappiness." It is temporal; it comes and goes and you cannot hold it, try as you will. This ephemeral happiness begets the need for additional happiness. And so you chase after it everywhere and in the course of your chasing you experience much unhappiness. Your situation is like that of the man who forgets that he has put a precious gem in his pocket. Thinking he has lost it, he travels far and wide to regain it. Because the gem is always with him, he could terminate his futile quest at any time that he put his hand in his pocket. In the same way, having forgotten that Self, Happiness, Bliss is your true nature, you seek it elsewhere. But it is always in your "pocket."

Student: It seems that most of the world is ignorant of this.

RH: Reintegrate yourself in your own Happiness and then you can turn your concern to the rest of the world.

Student: I find a great deal of happiness in my family and in my work.

RH: If your family and work were taken away, would your happiness go with them?

Student: Probably. Yes.

RH: And then you would need to find another family and other work in order to regain your happiness?

Student: I'm not sure.

RH: Then this cannot be the Happiness of Self. This Happiness has no coming and going and coming and going. This Happiness IS.

Another Student: How *should* we regard those whom we love?

RH: They cannot be loved in a personal, selective, particularized manner. You believe that you have a "self" that loves other "selves." This "love" that you speak of now appears to emanate from "you." Trace this love to its source and you will understand that there is not a "you" who loves "others." There is only LOVE.

Another Student: Speaking of having one's family "taken away," I would like to hear your comments on the death of loved ones. In the past two years I lost both my husband and a son. My son was only twenty-two. It has devastated me. I suffered intensely for many, many months and even now I don't see that I'll ever overcome the grief I still feel.

(This woman spoke falteringly and was obviously disturbed.)

RH: "Taken away" is only an expression; it has no reality. There is no place for your husband and son to be "taken" to. Your grief results from a sense of loss, but this loss rests entirely with you. Those who die experience no loss and are usually delighted to be rid of the body. The time had come for them to be out of the body and so they left it. They were not yours, that you may decide when they can be permitted to discard their bodies. You believe yourself to be confined in a physical body, so you extend this belief to include others: when their bodies die, you believe *they* have died. But what is eternal cannot die. All is eternal in Self. If you examine the situation carefully, you will understand that your grief arises entirely from *your* sense of deprivation. Investigate to determine *who* experiences this loss and your grief will dissolve.

Student: All right. I thank you. I've told myself some of the things you just said.

RH: You can't "tell yourself." "Telling yourself" is ordinary mind having a dialogue with ordinary mind. You must become one-pointed and go directly to the source of the *who*.

Student: Grief is a very strong emotion. I've never known suffering like that of the past two years.

RH: I also had a child who died at an early age. Do as I've suggested: continue to fix your mind on *who* it is that "knows suffering."

Another Student: How many children do you have?

RH: Five. Four boys and a girl.

Student: Do they all practice Yoga?

RH: The eldest, who is in his twenties, is a serious student. One is still too young, although he does the *asanas*. Three are only moderately interested, although they have been exposed to the teachings for some years now, and I think that their interest will increase as they grow older. Some of you have seen two of them in my television series.

Student: What is the best way to transmit these teachings to children?

RH: Introduce them to the asanas through the television programs or let them see you practicing. They may want to join you. If not, don't pressure them. If they're quite young, find interesting metaphysical story books through a metaphysical or regular bookstore. There are different series of such books that can usually be ordered. There are even metaphysical comic books that are imported from the Far East and present the material in an easily assimilated format. Speak to the youngsters about the adventure and fun of quieting the mind, and make a game of it: have them see if they can quiet their minds a few minutes each day. Meditate with them. In certain elementary schools in the Orient, this practice is a regular part of the daily curriculum.

Hatha Yoga and the various meditation practices are very "in" these days and teen-agers can usually be encouraged to experiment with them. Indeed, in numerous instances, it has been the young people who have introduced Yoga and related practices to their parents! Whenever appropriate, convey to them some of the things you are hearing and learning here. But all must be done with discrimination and you must be sensitive to what is required in a particular conversation or situation. Young people who are regularly exposed to the things we are practicing and discussing here will never forget them. They may not immediately react in an overt way, but they will retain far more than you may suspect. If your presentation of these techniques is sustained over a period of years, they are certain to become an important influence in the young person's life.

Another Student: You may recall that I'm a public-school teacher and that when I was here last year I told you of my plans to develop a number of Yoga programs in the school system where I teach. Well, to make a long story short, I'm happy to tell you that I've been successful and that we now have Yoga exercises and breathing included in several of our physical-education classes. The kids love it.

RH: Splendid! As I think most of you know, I believe that including this type of training is a great service to children. Long after they have lost interest in the various strenuous sports, they can continue to maintain their health and well-being through the Yoga routines they learned in in school. That is *real* education. Also, there would be much benefit derived from having the children engage in brief periods of sitting quietly, following the physical sessions.

Student: Yes, I'm doing a little of that with them now and I plan to do more.

Another Student: I met your little boy Joshua. He's a dear. Does he seem receptive to the Yoga teachings?

RH: It's difficult to judge what constitutes "receptivity" at the age of four. The other day I had occasion to tell him that who he really was, was not in his body. He thought this over a moment and replied, "If I'm not in my body, then I must be on the roof." This response was too profound for me and I dropped the subject.
   (Laughter)

Student: I would like to ask you about those who are born malformed. I have a relative who is the dearest, kindest person, but who, because of a birth defect, is paralyzed from the waist down. Is this her karma?

RH: Everything that occurs—past, present, and future—is "karma." What can befall a person, in the condition of *maya*, that would be outside karma? We accommodate the insatiable curiosity of ordinary mind through use of the word *karma*. This pulls it up short and momentarily halts its train of questions; the briefest respite from the conjurings of ordinary mind is to your advantage in the Yoga practice. The use of the word *karma* is, therefore, an expedient. But many think that *karma* is synonymous with *destiny*. Then, they want to know how they can control their destinies—as if one illusion can "control" another. Karma is not destiny. There is no Big Gambler in the sky who is rolling the dice to determine the course of your life. Karma is the doctrine of cause and effect. But if we begin to inquire which causes have which effects, and why should your relative, who is a dear and kind person, be afflicted with this paralysis, there will not only be no end to such inquiries, but the answers which will satisfy ordinary mind cannot be furnished. Once you understand this, you need no longer be concerned with karma. What good will it do you to be thinking always about karma—except to put an end to it? One can always turn the mind inward and rest in Self, regardless of one's physical condition. Frequently, those with serious physical handicaps gain a very direct understanding of the fact that one's true nature is not confined within the body.

Another Student: You say, "Turn inward." Where is "inward"?

RH: It is necessary that *you* find the place of the "inward." The "turning" is accomplished by introverting the ordinary mind and seeking the point at which the "I" thought arises. When you say, "*I* want to know . . ." *who* is this "I" and from *where* is it originating?

(Pause)

Who are you talking about when you say "Me"?

Student (Placing her hand on her chest): Me!

RH: Are you presenting your physical body as *you*? And when your body dies, as it most certainly will, will *you* also die?

Student: I don't know. I'm not sure.

RH: If you don't know that *you* are eternal—that you do not die, that you have not been born, and that what is eternal is not confined within the body—then it would be well for you to apply yourself toward this understanding.

Student: This is said to be the Age of Aquarius. Are more people involved in spiritual and metaphysical pursuits than in previous ages?

RH: We don't know about other ages. However, it is obvious that in the Western world, the great preoccupation with material acquisition has definitely decreased during the past decade—particularly on the part of the younger age groups. It is probable that interest in Eastern religion and philosophy is currently at an all-time high. Understand, however, that these historical speculations do not further your practice or insight. All such curiosities merely perpetuate ordinary mind and divert you from what must be done.

Another Student: I have a nephew who was going to law school and was going to practice law in his father's law firm when he graduated. He seemed to have a very secure future. Then he became interested in an Eastern sect—frankly, I've forgotten which one—and he dropped out of school and now he just spends his days walking around. His parents are heartbroken. They've been giving him money and they've threatened to stop that, but he says that he doesn't care. He just refuses to do anything. He's told his parents that they may believe he's not being functional, but that this is a part of the philosophy. What do you think about this?

RH: Well, he's young, and although you don't know what path he's following, it would be prudent to give him time to do what he must without harassment from his family. Young people often equate "doing nothing" with "freedom." Eventually, they learn otherwise. Freedom has nothing to do with the manner in which one's activities are structured or whether there is a renunciation of materialism. Freedom lies in recognition of Self and *only in this recognition*. However, at this time, you certainly will not be able to force him into returning to law school; he may do so of his own volition at a later time. But regardless of this, the main point to be noted here is that no Eastern philosophy or religion which is concerned with the doctrine of Self-recognition is a license for "dropping out," or for engaging in those activities which the society regards as immoral or illegal. If one wishes to be immoral, that is one thing. But if he interprets the philosophy or religion of which he claims to be an adherent as giving him license for this immorality, that is quite another thing.

His misinterpretation should be pointed out in no un-certain terms.

Another Student: Why? What is the difference between being immoral and being immoral under the guise of a philosophical persuasion?

RH: Because he may be thoroughly convinced that follow-ing the path that is dictated by this particular philoso-phy will lead to Self-recognition. But this objective will not be achieved unless the philosophy is correctly applied.

First Student: How can I explain this to my nephew?

RH: I cannot answer this. I don't know the man in ques-tion. You might relate to him what I've just said. Perhaps he will wish to reconsider his posture.

Another Student: But even if the incorrect means are used now, won't he eventually find the correct means? Won't we all eventually find the correct means?

RH: What is the sense of speaking about "eventually"? Do you mean one year? ten years? two lifetimes? a hundred lifetimes? NOW is when Self must manifest.

Student: There is a Chinese saying that if the wrong man uses the right means, the right means work in the wrong way.

RH: This is a riddle, a game for ordinary mind. There is no such thing as the "wrong man."

Student: If you have a guru and he dies, can he continue to guide you after his death?

RH: You do not understand who the guru is. You think of yourself as being confined in a body, so you see the guru as being confined in a body. Do you think that a "living," physical guru speaks from his body? And when his physical body decomposes, will he also de-compose? The guru is *always within*.

Student: How can you contact a guru or saint who is no longer in a physical form?

RH: Why would you want to do that?

Student: To be guided by him or her.

RH: You are already being guided in the most direct manner possible. Why do you require an intermediary? Listen for the guidance of the guru within.

Another Student: Why interpose *any* guru at all—either external *or* internal? Isn't this just creating another superfluous element? If Self is indivisible, why should we seek or consult a guru?

RH: As you say, Self is indivisible. The inner guru *is* Self. He is Self pulling you inward. Whenever you recognize that you ARE SELF NOW, you have no need of the guru or the concept of Self. But if your recognition of Self (Yoga) is not yet complete, without interruption, then continued guidance is necessary. The ordinary mind encourages you to seek guidance in all sorts of matters in the world. So we accommodate ordinary mind by inferring that guidance is also necessary for the *inner* journey and that it is the guru who guides. This concept is "rational" and must at least be *considered* by ordinary mind; it cannot be dismissed out-of-hand as "nonsense." In effect, we attempt to manuever the ordinary mind into a position where it must admit to a certain logic in seeking guidance from a guru, even if this guru is not immediately perceived. We continue to inform the ordinary mind that the inner guru *can* be found through certain techniques and, in this way, we may eventually prevail upon it to seek this inner guru—if only out of curiosity. The serious seeker soon learns, through his dedicated practice, that the guidance—the guru—takes the form of a force which pulls him inward toward the center. This guidance is subtle and sublime; it cannot be described, but it is unmistakable and ever-present. So either *jump* into the center NOW and abide there or *go within* and become receptive to the inner guidance of the guru.

Another Student: How do you "go within"?

RH: Go within the way you have come out. Retrace your steps.

Student: You have repeatedly told us that we are always Self. Therefore, we must already be "within."

RH: Of course. You [meaning the group] have been posing questions which indicate that you do not Know that one neither comes out nor goes in. If the ordinary mind represents you as being "out," then we must accommodate it by speaking in terms of going "within." Once recognizing that you neither come nor go, you have no further need of guidance, questions, or discussions. The man who is at home does not go out in the street and ask those who pass by for directions to his house. I believe it was the philosopher Pascal who said something about all of man's difficulties arising because he is unable to sit home quietly in his study. This observation holds something of value for the aspirant: when the mind is perceived to be flowing outward, getting you involved in all sorts of trouble by both fabricating and solving "problems," reel it in and have it sit quietly in its study.

Student: If people never went out into the world, nothing could be accomplished.

RH: You persist in your belief that ordinary mind is responsible for "accomplishing" and that *you* are the one who "acts" and "does." The truth is that All is Self. ALL IS without the illusion of ordinary mind. When your car is up on the rack in the service station, do you run beneath it and put your arms up to help support it? Not only is there no necessity for such support from you, but if the car were to fall, your arms would be useless as support. In the same way is the ordinary mind extraneous. ALL does not require that anything be "accomplished."

Student: And a person would not become a vegetable without his mind?

RH: Is the existence of the magician dependent on the illusion he creates? Does he vanish when the illusion vanishes? Only when you recognize that the ordinary mind is an illusion can you truly *experience*. You are a "vegetable" if you do not experience as Self. As long as the ordinary mind is a reality, you exist in a subject-object relationship with all things. You never EXPERIENCE and you never KNOW.

Student: If ordinary mind is an illusion, how can you turn it inward?

RH: As long as it appears real to you, you must turn it inward. It is in the turning inward that its illusory nature is revealed.

Another Student: I can't understand how our everyday problems—all the things we have to cope with every minute—can be properly dealt with if the mind is not active.

RH: In what you call your "everyday life," you see yourself beset with continual "problems." These problems appear to be external to you—that is, they appear to be caused by people, circumstances and events that are apart from you. What you are failing to recognize—and what the ordinary mind is utterly ingenious in camouflaging—is that *the very entity that appears to be solving the problems is the entity that is also creating the problems*! There are no problems apart from ordinary mind. The nature of the ordinary mind is that of conceptualization: it invents endless problems and then pretends to be your loyal servant and ally by undertaking to "solve" these problems. It is like the unscrupulous exterminator who, as he sprays his poisons throughout the house to kill the insects, simultaneously plants the eggs that will hatch new insects so that his services will be required again. There can be no end to your problems unless there is an end to the problem maker—ordinary mind.

Another Student: The more you consider the situation, the more strange it becomes! I mean that ordinary mind, which is in itself an illusion, can distort our true nature to the extent that we completely believe ourselves to be something that we are totally and absolutely *not*!

RH: Well said.

(Pause)

Do you recall the Hall of Mirrors in the amusement park? You are startled as each mirror in turn distorts your image in a different way. You are reflected as short and fat, tall and thin, upside down, and so forth. You laugh because you know that these are *distortions* and they do not reflect the way you *really* appear. In the same way, as Self, you laugh at the various distortions which the ordinary mind, the ego, has assumed: it has projected a good I, a bad I, an I who can be right and an I who can be wrong, an I who cherishes diversity and possibilities, an I who quests for happiness while it simultaneously contrives to avoid sorrow, and a myriad of other I's. As Self, you laugh at these manifold distortions of Self because you Know that none of these reflections is You.

Student: Yes, I understand. It's an incredible trick of the mind!

RH: The ordinary mind is itself the "trick." It is the ultimate "con man." It fabricates the "Big Store" (the world), and "cons" you into believing that you can place your bets there and win (find your happiness, security, and fulfillment). The *ultimate* "mark" is the man who swallows the story that he can even find him*self* there. No one is more of a "sucker" than he who says, "I am trying to *find* myself!" The conspirators laud this man in his noble search for "self" and "meaning," but he can no more find himself in the world than the donkey can catch the carrot which is tied on a stick and held by the rider before the donkey's eyes to entice him into moving. The carrot moves at the exact rate of speed as does the donkey. The self can never catch up with the self. No one can "find" his self. He need only recognize his true nature—that of Self!

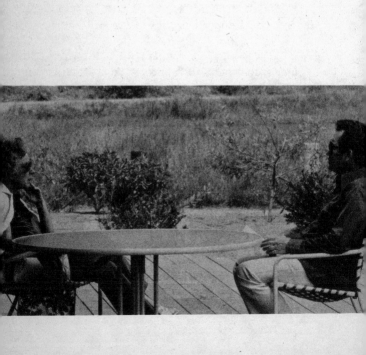

5th day

Student: This is something you touched on the other day, about families. I can't tell you how much the Yoga postures and the meditation have meant to me. Well, I know I don't have to say anything about it because you understand. I couldn't get my husband interested in Hatha Yoga even though it would be very beneficial for him, but at one point he was attracted to meditation. I explained whatever I could to him and he joined me in a few practice sessions. Then he stopped. He said that his mind was just "too active," and that he was "too motivated" by the world to be able to withdraw his mind from it. I felt badly about this. I wasn't sure how to reply to him at that time, but I've learned many important things from these meetings and perhaps I can arouse his interest again. I thought you might give me some additional advice.

RH: Well, you see how his ordinary mind rationalized its own disturbance: the uncontrollable movement was attributed to being "too motivated." He accepted this phrase about "motivation" as a satisfactory explanation. Then he felt justified in dismissing the entire matter. His ordinary mind perceived the threat and dispatched it quickly with a few well-chosen phrases. But what does "motivation" mean? It is a synonym for "desire." The ordinary man accepts motivations and desires without much question, as the natural course of events. Indeed, the society (the conspiracy) condones motivation and applauds one who is *highly* motivated. In truth, desire is *not* natural; it is a disease. The stronger the desires, the more serious the illness. Desire begets desire without end and the fever will not abate. A person infected with desire cannot know peace.

The ordinary man does not know the source of his desires. From time to time he may question the *types* of desires he is entertaining and he may evaluate them as "healthy" or "destructive," but he never questions the *nature of desire itself*. Where do desires come from? Why does he think them "natural"? If he seriously sought the answers to these questions, he would begin to understand how his desires confine him permanently in the prison of his ordinary mind, where he experiences no peace. If, when you perceive a desire arising—and it is entirely possible to cultivate such perception—you become quiet for a few moments and attempt to "feel" its nature, "feel" what is transpiring throughout your body and mind, you will recognize the disturbance that is manifesting. The stronger the desire, the more intense the disturbance. And these disturbances intense and less intense, are occurring incessantly, like waves in the ocean. Now, observe the folly inherent in the situation: a man is "highly motivated," which means that his ordinary mind drives him mercilessly into the world and convinces him that there he can gratify his desires. He may, indeed, be able to gratify certain desires, but in the course of his efforts to do so, myriad *new* desires are generated. The time never arrives when he is able to say, "There, that's it! I've satisfied my last desire. Now I'm finished and I can relax in peace." The irony is that he is involved in all this gratification of desire so that he can know peace and security, but the nature of desire is to spawn additional desire, so there can be no peace.

Another Student: What is the solution?

RH: Find out where the desires come from.

Student: Is this the same as turning the mind inward?

RH: Yes. If you penetrate to that place from which the ego arises, you will understand how to still desires. Desires arise from the ego, from the thought of "I," because it is the "I" that demands aggrandizement. So, by introverting the ordinary mind, turning it inward, backward, or however you wish to conceive the practice of sense and thought withdrawal from the external world, disturbances are terminated.

Student: Permanently?

RH: It depends upon the degree of penetration. Practice seriously and regularly, and you will understand what is involved soon enough.

Another Student: What about the desires of the body— hunger, thirst, sleep, and so forth?

RH: These are natural requirements of the organism, not desires of the ordinary mind for aggrandizement of an illusory "self." The distinction is evident.

Student: What about the sexual desire?

RH: Each must resolve this according to his or her level of understanding. Those who have taken vows of continence understand the nature of these vows. This is a form of self-surrender. Those who do not observe continence should elevate their sexual relations above sensuality to the symbolic act of terminating duality. There are sects in India which ritualize the sexual act: each of the participants regards the partner as an aspect of

Self. In this way, each *merges* with Self and the act becomes what may be called "spiritual" rather than carnal. Of course, each of the participants must be knowledgeable in the dynamics of his and her role in this act.

Another Student: Various Yogic scriptures prohibit sex.

RH: Yes, to those who are unmarried and have dedicated themselves to spiritual practices along very well-defined lines; not to those who are "householders," who are married or who are living with another, married or not.

Student: Certain texts, addressed to the male student, state very specifically that strength and resolve are weakened through loss of semen.

RH: This may be the case for those who have dedicated their lives to Hatha Yoga and certain other practices. It need not be a factor in turning the mind inward and other forms of meditation.

Student: What about homosexuality or sexual acts that society currently labels "abnormal"?

RH: All can turn their minds inward.

Student: So there are no sex regulations that you consider mandatory?

RH: Only moderation, to avoid enervation that detracts from one's ability to practice seriously and regularly. It is meaningless to impose other regulations in this extremely personal matter. Such things become known through practice and meditation. The dedicated student is not left in the dark as to the most expedient course for him to follow.

Student: What if one finds it very difficult to observe moderation? What if he or she experiences a continual and overpowering urge for sex?

RH: I assume, of course, that in these questions you are always speaking about the student, about one who is involved in practice. That student should turn the mind inward and find the place from *where* this urge is originating. In this investigation, the urge subsides. Also, such urges, which are of a gross nature, can be channeled into the practice of Hatha Yoga, where they will be refined. This refined energy is then utilized, to very good advantage, in the practice of meditation.

Another Student: But don't you need to have "desire" in order to turn the mind inward and to practice Yoga?

RH: We've discussed this previously and I believe you were here. As various desires arise, you can transform them by channeling them all into one desire—that which you just mentioned: the desire to turn the mind inward and to practice. However, as you continue your serious practice, that which was formerly the *desire* to practice now becomes your *way of life*, free of desire.

Another Student: I want to get this straight again. I grasp it while we are talking here, but when I think about it later it often slips away. If we quiet our desire or motivation, won't our lives be drastically changed—for all the obvious reasons?

RH: What is the basic purpose of one's efforts to gratify his desires? It is that of Self-revelation. No matter how far afield your desires and motivations appear to take you, in everything you do you are seeking restoration in Self. The desire for success in business, love, school, and in all the countless other ventures that people undertake, is fundamentally the desire for permanent happiness, security, and peace. Examine your desires and your activities and you will find that the quest for Self is at the bottom of all. So why do you wish to perpetuate desires which will compel you to engage in interminable activities—through as many lifetimes as there are grains of sand on the beaches? Why not respose in Self NOW and put an end to these futile endeavors which are the causes of your vexation?

Student: But if all desires eventually lead you to Self, they're not really "futile."

RH: What would you think about someone in this room who desperately wanted to go down to the beach— which is about two hundred yards from where we are sitting—and went there by way of Chicago?

Student: Pretty dumb!

RH: Precisely! Why travel the "eventual" route when you're but a stone's throw away from your destination? Attain your liberation from desire *now*.

Another Student: What about an archfiend and mass murderer such as Hitler? Were his nefarious exploits also undertaken in the search for Self?

RH: All search for Self who do not recognize that they *are* Self. Hitler's illusion was that ultimate fulfillment lay in a particular type of *power*. Because of the monumental scale on which he sought this power and the methods he implemented to gain it, his illusion is pointed up in a very direct way. But you must understand, also, the nature of your own illusions.

RH: I'd like to mention a few points which came up in my consultations with students last night because I believe they are relevant to the group as a whole. First, regarding drugs that alter the consciousness or awareness: you cannot practice Yoga and meditation, and indulge in drug experiences. As you probably know, there are very few things I tell you that, without qualification, you cannot do. But drugs present a very real and constant danger. Not only is there the physical danger— and we'll let this pass for now because that danger is a matter of degree, according to what you're taking—but there are two other dangers which are, perhaps, even more serious. First, drugs weaken your ability to practice as is necessary. They enervate you physically, so that proper Hatha Yoga practice is impeded; the lungs and the nervous and circulatory systems are impaired. If any of you are attempting to minimize or dismiss this weakening property of drugs, you are making a grave error. Then, too, the steadiness, balance, and one-

---

pointedness necessary for correct meditation are equally impaired by "pot," "uppers" and "downers," LSD, hashish, cocaine, heroin, and whatever else is currently in vogue.

Second, and perhaps the greatest danger, is that you may come to believe that the drug experience is somehow akin to Self-awareness. This is not the case. The drug "high" is not the experience of Pure Consciousness; it is counterfeit. Each time the user gets high, his awareness is altered in a way that usually seems very desirable. Consequently, he begins to think, "Meditation requires dedication and effort. Why expend such effort when I can smoke a 'joint,' shoot some 'H,' sniff some 'C,' take a pill, eat an LSD sugar cube. . . ." And so either he never undertakes practice, or his practice is weak, or he starts and stops and starts and stops and can never really make progress, or he simply has to abandon practice altogether. Then, too, there is the very real fact of the impermanence of all such drug highs. When the user is "on," he may feel and speak of love, God, beauty, and so forth. Not only is he *not* experiencing the Reality of such things, but soon he is once again "down," and *then* where is his love and beauty? He needs to get high again; he's "hooked" on an illusion, on what is just another aspect of the not-Self. So, *that* is the danger: the user has not only mistaken the unreal for the Real, but, to a very great extent, he weakens his ability for undertaking that practice which *can* result in Self-consciousness. Therefore, those of you who are serious about our work here, and who may be inclined to indulge in drugs—even for what you consider only an occasional "kick"—must absolutely put an end to this inclination. Understand that through the use of drugs your consciousness cannot be "raised" or "expanded" in any way which is significant in our work. The permanent transformation of consciousness occurs only in Self-recognition.

Another Student: Is the same true for alcohol?

RH: Yes, in every detail—with the possible exception that alcohol is almost always a direct and immediate "downer." That is, you don't even have the illusion of the consciousness being "raised." Feeling happy, jolly, uninhibited, gregarious, and those other emotions that may be evoked through alcohol and are considered desirable—in contrast to depression, hostility, and physical illness, which may also result—have no advantage whatsoever in relation to our work. Also, of course, meditating while under the influence of alcohol is impossible.

Student: What about moderate indulgence that is sometimes necessary in business and social situations?

RH: Do what you must do. There is no situation in which introducing alcohol, an unquestionably harmful chemical, into the organism cannot be avoided. If you drink, it's because you want to.

Another Student: What about wine?

RH: I believe I've made the point. Do what you must do.

Another Student: Hasn't the practice of Yoga been very helpful to many drug addicts? I've heard that in some cases Yoga and meditation are the only things that were really effective.

Another Student: I personally know of a number of therapy programs for addicts that include the Yoga practices—breathing, meditation, and so forth.

RH: Yes.

Student: Have you had experience with such programs?

RH: Yes, but we needn't discuss these things at this time.
  (Pause)
  Are there any other comments on this point?
  (There were none.)
  Then, a few words about another matter that came up last night. One of the Yoga teachers who is here for our Teacher's Seminar told me that a number of stu-

dents had come to her when their teacher was no longer available. It seems that these students were full of the "glamour" and "excitement" of studying Yoga. Apparently, their teacher had imbued them with her personal, diversionary fantasies of what was involved in the practice: the acquisition of ESP, astral bodies, secret initiations, gaining the unbounded admiration of their friends, and lots and lots of success in all their undertakings. In other words, the practice of Yoga was "romanced" like a lipstick commercial. Now, I've been involved in similar situations. Publishers have written promotional copy for my books and television promos have been made regarding my programs which reflect this same romantic and unknowledgeable conception. The rationale for this is that people are seeking to improve and aggrandize their "selves" and are frequently attracted to Yoga on this basis. Also, as we know, the promise of magic powers, secret doctrines, and so forth holds a strong attraction for many. So, there are extenuating circumstances for utilizing this romance, adventure, and intrigue approach, because from the viewpoint of the ordinary mind the Yogas do improve health, promote well-being and longevity, and impart insight into dimensions of life that are generally obscured. A very significant number of people have begun their practice of Yoga with these superficial objectives and have gone on to become serious students of Hatha, Jnana, and Raja. The point I wish to make here is that the instructor of a Yoga class or a small group of private students is not in the situation of promoting a book or planning the format for a television series which must be presented to accommodate the level of understanding of several million people. It is possible that this teacher will attract her students on the basis of self-improvement, but early on in that class the more profound objectives of Yoga practice should be clearly stated. Those in the class who are seeking glamour, excitement, adventure, power, recognition, success, or who are in attendance simply to have something about which to talk to their friends, should not be encouraged in such pursuits, but rather should be informed of their illusory nature. If the teacher is unable to convey this clearly, she does her students a disservice and her qualifications as an instructor of Yoga should be questioned. So, I tell those of you who may be harboring similar illusions to discard them. The serious student practices without discussing her practice with others, without looking for "results" or "progress," by observing "visions" or whatever else she witnesses with dispassion, and without any need or desire to utilize the powers [*siddhis*] which she may acquire. Those who envision the path as a series of satisfying "accomplishments" are still prisoners of their ordinary minds and may regard what I have just said as disappointing. But those whose quest is for uncompromising liberation will recognize that these principles of silence, balance, and dispassion comprise the true Way.

Student: I assume you're not in favor of astrology.

RH: How does it relate to you?

Student: I've had my horoscope cast for many years by one of the foremost astrologers in the country, and I've found it very helpful in directing my efforts into certain channels at particular times.

RH: What has this to do with recognition of your true nature? Is there ever a "particular time" at which you are unable to turn your mind inward?

Student: No, I believe not. But I might do this to better advantage at certain times than at others.

RH: Nonsense! The serious student cannot permit herself to be influenced by such things. You and all the celestial bodies whose movements you believe can somehow "influence" you are Self. The life that you believe is yours is actually unconditioned existence which springs spontaneously, each moment, as Self. It IS complete and cannot be "influenced" in any manner whatsoever. You ARE Self. You are not an individual self living a life—like a train running along a track—which can be influenced by external conditions. As Self, you are totally complete and unchanging. Having your horoscope cast and consulting it to determine how and where your efforts should be directed will perpetuate your illusion that you are a separate self, vulnerable to the whims of destiny and fate, and you will be driven to all sorts of devices in a futile attempt to stay out in front of your life, to get "one up" on what may influence it. Put an end to all these illusions now. Recognize your eternal ONENESS.

Another Student: I see. There's no point in attempting to predict what the future may hold.

RH: What future? What would you do with a "future"? Is it not enough that you ARE ETERNALLY NOW?

Another Student (After a pause): But the future allows you to have hope.

RH: Hope for what? You are already fulfilled. You have never been unfulfilled, that you require hope. Hope is the opiate held out by the conspirators, like the carrot in front of the donkey, and it is one of their most powerful and cherished illusions. It promises: what you do not *now* have you can *someday* have, providing you undertake the proper mayic activities. But "someday" never comes because it always remains an idea. So, by continually conjuring up this ingenious diversion of "hope," ordinary mind effectively circumvents your immediate and direct recognition of the fact that you ARE SELF NOW. Thus, ordinary mind is able to hypnotize you with anticipation and send you on a perpetual "wild goose chase": you entertain the illusory "hope" of finding illusory "fulfillment" in an illusory "future." Now, that's *really* self-deception.

Student: I don't think many people could stand having hope taken away from them.

RH: Hope is not given and it is not taken away. It is an illusion which is inherent in a fabricated "future." Ordinary mind will appear to indulge you in exposing many of its deceptions, even those which are insidious and ruthless. But when you dare to question "hope," ordinary mind evokes the emotion of rage. This is one dis-illusionment it attempts to prevent at all costs. As you said, millions live by hope. Everyone wants to be fulfilled, and if you are unaware that you are fulfilled NOW, then your fulfillment seems possible only in a "future." You may even be convinced that Self-recognition will occur at some future time. Therefore, any questioning, any close scrutiny of the concept of hope, is made strictly taboo by the ordinary mind. "Hands off of hope," it warns. But the Yoga student *must* awaken from the hypnotic spell of hope. You must see its nature clearly, because you cannot recognize that you are Self, NOW, when you are "hoping" that this recognition will occur in an imagined "future." "Hope" is characterized by the conspirators as something that is noble and beautiful: "All mankind must have hope," they declare. This idea is so effective in diverting one from the real business at hand that they make certain it is reiterated at every turn: you are encouraged to "hope" for anything and everything in a nonexistent future!

Student: But what about the sick who have hope of recovery, the poor who have hope of improving their situation, and so forth?

RH: All is NOW. You ARE Self. Recognize your true nature as Self and you will no longer have to deal with hope in any form. Do what you must do for the sick and the poor, but don't neglect to determine *who* it is that is concerned with their welfare.

Another Student: There are those who are less "hopeful" and more fatalistic. They live by the philosophy of "what will be, will be."

RH: The optimism of hope and the resignation of fatalism are both involved with an illusory future. Nothing "will be." There is no "present" that evolves into a "future." All IS. ALL IS NOW.

Another Student: You seem to be eliminating everything around which my life has been built!

RH: You do not "build" your life. Your existence is spontaneous; it is the ordinary mind that develops a past-present-future sequence and convinces you that what your life is in the so-called present is dependent on what you have "done" in the illusory "past." Have you ever existed, have you ever been aware, in any place or at any time other than NOW? Your illusion is not only that you "build" your life—like an engineer builds a bridge—but that you build it "around" other things. You say that I am "eliminating" these illusions, these other things, but that is not possible. If we should undertake to eliminate these other things, there will be no end to our work because there are no end to these "things." Ordinary mind will always dredge up more "things" around which it will encourage you to "build your life." All this "building" is a dream from which you must awaken. Since it is impossible to eliminate the "things" one by one, you must extinguish that which is the *source* of the "things." "Cut off the serpent's head with one blow." Then you will Know that you do not "build" your life and that there is no need for you to be endlessly concerned with attempting to protect this illusory structure.

Student: How do I "cut off its head"?

RH: Find out *who* it is that thinks she "builds" her life. Through this inward turning of the mind you reach the source of the illusion.

Student: Should you *prepare* the mind before you begin to ask "Who?"—or before you practice any other meditation? I mean, do you first perform the postures and then the breathing and then withdraw the senses and so forth before you begin the inquiry?

RH: It depends on the level of your meditation. Beginning students usually find it helpful, but not essential, to undertake the preliminaries you mentioned. These preliminaries aid in "rendering the consciousness fit for meditation." More-advanced students are *always* practicing meditation—whether it be the inward turning of the mind or another form—regardless of their external circumstances.

Another Student: If you continue to ask "Who?" how can the mind be quiet?

RH: It is quiet in the sense that it is "fixed" without distraction. It ceases to flow outward. We do not attempt to stupefy or numb the consciousness, but to center it, to hold it on the object of meditation. In this practice, "who" or "where" becomes the object.

Student: But then you have the subject-object relationship again.

RH: Fixing the consciousness on the object of meditation and remaining there with steady awareness effects a *mergence*. The one who is inquiring "Who?" merges with the "who" which is the object of the inquiry. At this point both "whos" dissolve and Self IS.

Student: But they may arise again?

RH: The *illusion* of the "whos" may remanifest, depending upon the strength or tendency [*vasana*] of the ordinary mind to pull outward. This illusion is like the waves of the ocean, which rise and take a temporary form but are never apart from the ocean. The ordinary mind manifests the illusion that there is an "I" that is inquiring about a "who." In Reality, both whos are always Self, just as the waves are always the ocean. The recognition of this Reality becomes permanent when ordinary mind is quieted to the extent that it no longer pulls outward. This ordinary mind, the maker of illusions, becomes quiescent through being continually turned inward and exposed to the illumination of Self.

Student: You said something about "recognition of Reality." Who is the one that is left to "recognize"?

RH: There is never, at any time, "recognition," because there is no one to do the "recognizing." These are words that we use to accommodate ordinary mind. Self IS. There is only eternal AWARENESS. You see what is involved here: your ordinary mind is now asking questions about a state in which it does not exist. Therefore, either there can be no response whatsoever, or we must reply in terms that will accommodate ordinary mind. As long as you continue this type of questioning—no matter how subtle or gross—we shall inevitably come to that point where we now find ourselves, where we can go no further. Each time we arrive at this point, the absolute necessity of *practice* is reinforced. This is the underlying theme of these discussions: to repeatedly bring ordinary mind to that point where it must admit that it is a limiting entity and can never Know Self. Through this admission we can turn it—the ordinary mind—to practice.

Student: You say that questioning is futile. What about the inquiry "who?"

RH: This is not a question to activate ordinary mind. It is one that leads to the extinguishment of ordinary mind. It is not asked in order that a conceptual response may be forthcoming. It is asked to direct the consciousness to that point *where* the question itself arises, and to discover *who* is asking it.

Student: Can other forms of meditation accomplish the same objective?

RH: Discovering the source of the ego, of that place from where it arises, is the most direct method of Self-recognition. But in the event that the student has difficulty with the "Who?" meditation, he may choose any other meditation technique which attracts him and which he finds easy. As you know, you are being instructed in a variety of techniques here for this very reason. Through these techniques, the phantom nature of the ordinary mind is exposed more gradually, but eventually the result will be the same.*

* These techniques have been incorporated into *Richard Hittleman's 30 Day Yoga Meditation Plan.* Bantam Books, New York, 1978.

Student: Does the practice of Yoga make you less sensitive to pain?

RH: In what way does this relate to you?

Student: Well, I've heard that Yogis are able to control their senses so that they do not feel pain. I would like to learn this.

RH: Under certain conditions, in which the senses are withdrawn, pain can be minimized or eliminated. But this is not within the exclusive domain of Yogis. Fakirs who lie on the "bed of nails" or walk on hot coals or cut glass have mastered this type of sense "withdrawal." Anyone may learn it through sufficient practice. Those who are seriously practicing Yoga are generally uninterested in cultivating withdrawal for this specific purpose, although such insensitivity may manifest as a by-product of their practice.

Another Student: Does the "liberated" person [*jnani*] feel pain?

RH: He may or may not. It depends upon the circumstances. According to accounts, Jesus and Ramakrishna suffered greatly—one in being crucified, the other from cancer. Other accounts tell of saints who displayed no evidence of pain even when subjected to torture. But you must understand that the experience of pain is not the same for the saint or liberated being as it is for the ordinary man. The ordinary man resists pain; he evaluates it as something alien, abnormal, undesirable, something to be avoided or eliminated. But the *jnani* experiences All, including pain, as Self. Therefore, what you now regard as "pain" is something of an entirely different nature in the enlightened condition.

Student: Do *you* [indicating RH] feel pain?

RH: Pain is "painful" as long as it is regarded from the point of view of self, which believes that Self is confined in and limited to a body. Therefore, put an end to all that is of the not-Self, and these curiosities of the ordinary mind—such as whether I or others experience pain—will no longer divert you.

Another Student: Isn't pain an important indication that something requires attention in the body?

RH: Of course. This is for the sake of the body. It in no way alters what I have said.

Student: But if pain is disregarded, a serious condition might develop.

RH: Nothing was said about "disregarding" pain. You believe Self to be confined to your body; therefore, your preoccupation with the body is almost total. Recognize Self and your experience of body and pain will be very different than it is now.

Student: Certain drugs render the body insensitive to pain.

RH: A temporary expedient. This numbness has nothing to do with Self-recognition.

Another Student: If loss of the sense of being in a body is an objective, why practice Hatha Yoga, which emphasizes the reality of the body?

RH: Your question is asked from the point of view of ordinary mind, not from the unconditioned perspective of Self. No sense of "loss" occurs, only recognition that you have never been limited to a body. Hatha Yoga is concerned only superficially with health and well-being. Its major objective is to disclose to the practitioner that he is *not* confined to the body. Hatha Yoga is that most marvelous method of utilizing the body to discover the nature of the body. In discovering the nature of the body, one can discover All.

Student: If Self can be uncovered through the body, then Self must be *in* the body.

RH: This premise is acceptable, in Yoga, as a starting point for practice. It is a theory that accomodates ordinary mind. But the Self's true relation to the body is discerned in the course of serious Hatha practice.

Student: What is the purpose of existence?

RH: Why must existence have a "purpose"?

Student: Everything has some purpose.

RH: "Purpose" is an illusion of ordinary mind. *Nothing* has any "purpose." Because of the way in which ordinary mind regards the elements of the world—as influencing and affecting one another—it concludes that these relationships must be "purposeful," that something must result from their doing what they are doing, that something else must result from that result, and so on forever. It goes so far as to imply that someday, when enough "facts" have been uncovered by the researchers, we will at last know the "purpose" of life. Of course, no such time will ever arrive, because "purpose" and "time" are inventions of the ordinary mind. There will always be more "facts" to uncover, more "discoveries" to be made.

You may wish to fabricate a "purpose" for your life, your activities, or whatever; you can even fabricate *many* purposes for each of these. But even a little serious reflection will disclose that none of these are based on Reality. None ring True. The ordinary mind is dismayed and rebels when you challenge its cherished twins, "purpose" and "hope." "If there's no purpose," it whines, "then what's it all for anyhow?" But as you continue to meditate you will understand—and this understanding will bring about a great relief and happiness—that it is not "for" anything! Existence, Awareness, IS. You ARE. Isn't that purpose enough? Could there be any more significant purpose?

Another Student (After a pause): Then you could say that the purpose of existence is to find out that there is no purpose.

RH: Yes, you could say that if you want to go to the beach by way of Chicago. Why this circuitous route? Why subject yourself to the agony and torment of countless lifetimes dedicated to "finding out" what is meaningless? Why not simply Know that NOW?

Another Student: There are untold millions of people who believe that God has a plan for His creation.

RH: So you insist that there is a "creation" and that "God" is responsible for it. Very well, let us assume that is the case. Because the ordinary mind conceives and attempts to implement endless "plans" for self-gratification, this activity is made to be anthropomorphic and is imputed to the Absolute. What egocentricity, what presumption! A "plan" is subject to success and failure. Do you think that God, the Absolute, is of the nature of success and failure? Do you think that He "works out" plans in a space-time continuum? There is no "plan" and no "purpose." No plan was conceived at some point in the past, no plan is now "working out" in the present, and no plan will be concluded at some point in the future. All always IS.

Student (After a pause): Then there is no reason to do anything!

RH: You make this statement because you think that you are the doer. Find out *who* it is that acts and you will Know that there is no choice of "doing" or "not doing."

Student: If I believe that there is no point to life, I might be inclined not to care what happens or what I do.

RH: "Believe," "point," "purpose"—all fantasies! At this time, when you admittedly know nothing of what you call the "purpose" of life, do you not care what happens or what you do?

Student: No, I do care. But that may be because I hope that someday I *will* know.

RH: So, you see we are going around in a circle. I have just told you what you indicate you are willing to spend an infinite number of lifetimes in learning: there is no "purpose." But what you are now saying is that you really don't want to know this, because then you won't want to continue the search. Do you begin to understand the cunning, imprisoning nature of ordinary mind?

Student: Yes. I think I've been playing the devil's advocate in a number of the questions I've asked, because I *do* want to bang the teachings into my head so that they stay there.

(Laughter)

Another Student: With reference to "purpose" and "plan": How do you regard such theories as Evolution and the Expanding Universe?

RH: Self does not evolve or expand. These theories are spawned by ordinary mind, which appears to seek "answers" to the questions it, itself, has invented. The ordinary mind functions in terms of space and time and is always changing; consequently, all its theories evolve in space and time and must also change. What is the use of a "theory" to one who wants to KNOW? Does a decade pass in which new discoveries in the "sciences" do not alter the theories of the previous decade? With each pertinent discovery, the ordinary mind dramatically announces to the world that a "major breakthrough" has been made. But soon we begin to see that there is no end to these. The nature of the ordinary mind is to make "major breakthroughs" while simultaneously increasing the magnitude of the "problem," of what is yet "unknown." The ordinary mind lures you into examining the universe. To what end? Such an examination can never be satisfactorily concluded because each "breakthrough" will generate a multitude of new "unknowns." The scientist or researcher says, "Wonderful! These unknowns are the challenge and adventure of life for me." Very well. Let *him* investigate as he wishes. But for the Yoga student, only *direct* perception, absolute KNOWLEDGE, can suffice. This absolute Knowledge is revealed through abandoning the not-True for the True, the un-Real for the Real. The ordinary mind impedes direct and absolute perception. Therefore, The Yogi remains unpreoccupied with "theories."

Another Student: What if one who is in a scientific field takes a serious interest in Yoga? How can he reconcile the Yoga teachings with his work?

RH: Let us not concern ourselves with hypothetical matters. Are you speaking about yourself?

Student: My husband.

RH: All such conflicts are resolved for practicing Yogis. Problems dissolve and illusions vanish through the force generated by their practice. One need make no elaborate psychological preparations or change his vocation to begin Yoga. All will be reconciled of its own accord in the course of serious practice.

Student: Does it help our practice to study and read about Yoga and Vedanta? If so, what do you recommend?

RH: You will receive a bibliography of basic works at this seminar. [*Editor's note: see bibliography at the end of this book.*] However, I advise only moderate reading. Many students who become "addicted" to reading begin to mistake their intellectual comprehension of the doctrine for the direct perception of it. Students of Eastern religions and philosophies often commit an enormous quantity of technical information to memory—Sanskrit and Buddhist terms, structures of systems, comparisons—and they engage in a great deal of conjecture as to interpretation of doctrines. Most of this diverts one from *practice* and is what Ramana Maharshi characterized as "learned ignorance." Self cannot be found in the written word. Reading of the scriptures and other pertinent works should serve as an external "push" for practice and should not become a diversion or a substitute for practice. If you ever find that you are neglecting your practice because of excessive reading, make the necessary adjustments.

Student: I know that you think highly of fasting. How does fasting relate to meditation?

RH: There is no direct connection. One may often meditate to advantage during a fast, but the student should not make meditation dependent upon fasting. The suggested *sattvic* [spiritually helpful] diet of light, easily digested, natural foods will facilitate meditation. There is no doubt that a direct connection does exist, especially for the beginning student, between one's diet and one's ability to hold his mind fixed and steady. Flesh foods, rich, spicy, greasy, heavy foods, and drinks that overly stimulate, disturb, or congest the organism should be consumed very moderately or, preferably, eliminated entirely. It is a simple matter for the student to experiment with the sattvic diet and determine its advantages, not only in terms of health but as it relates to meditation practice. The meals that you are being served here at the workshop are totally sattvic. My various books on nutrition deal in detail with the suggested diet.

Student: May I ask how long *you* fast?

RH: Twice a year I fast for approximately thirty days. In addition, I fast intermittently during the year for one to two weeks each time. I do this for purposes of cleansing and resting the organism, not as a punitive measure or to precipitate a change in consciousness. One should understand his reasons for fasting and feel psychologically at ease in doing it.

Another Student: Certain texts and teachers advise against fasting.

RH: Each student must make the determination of what best furthers his practice. You must not undertake any practice we have been discussing solely on the basis that I or any other teacher has suggested it. Only if you feel a particular practice or teaching to be truthful and compelling should it be applied.

Another Student: Is this "feeling" immediate? I mean, do you know right away that a particular practice or teaching is appropriate?

RH: It can be an immediate attraction or it may be delayed;

it may need to "ripen" within you. The guru within guides. It is he who governs your attraction in these matters.

Another Student: I noticed that you were using the words *reasons* and *psychological* and other ordinary-mind concepts.

RH: If instruction is to be conveyed verbally in these matters, there are two ways to respond to ordinary mind: accommodate it or turn it back upon itself so that its assertions are invalidated. In the instruction of *techniques*, I almost always accommodate it because, paradoxically, the correct application of these techniques results in the dissolution of self, the transcendence of ordinary mind.

Student: How can a teacher continue to instruct about the non-Self once he has Self-recognition? How is it he can continue to perceive illusion and discuss it?

RH: Consider the case of a drug addict or an alcoholic who experiences dreadful hallucinations. Eventually, he breaks his addiction, recovers his health, and is no longer subject to these hallucinations. But when he encounters another man who is under the influence of drugs and alcohol and is suffering from hallucinations, he is able to assist this man because he vividly recalls the hallucinatory experience. He need no longer hallucinate to know what the second man is experiencing and how he is suffering. He does not need to hear the second man describe the details of his particular horrors because he knows the nature of the state in which the second man is dwelling. In the same way, one who has recovered his true nature can assist one who still dwells and suffers in the illusory state, without himself abiding there.

Student: Is death also an illusion?

RH: Yes. Death is envisioned by the ordinary man as the absence of life, as the opposite of life. But Self does not live and it does not die. It IS.

Student: So we continue to exist when the body dies?

RH: What is your understanding of "existence"?

Student: To be. That which is.

RH: And what about that which is *not*?

Student: I don't understand the question.

RH: Now consider this carefully: Self is beyond that which exists and that which does not exist. It is beyond what is and what is not. In attempting to convey to you that Self is beyond all duality, I say, "Self IS. You ARE." You see, I always place a very obvious emphasis on those words. [*Editor's note: Mr. Hittleman is referring here to those words which, in this book, appear fully capitalized or which have the first letter capitalized.*] The stress or emphasis on this word is to indicate that it has no opposite. When I say, "Recognize Self," I do not mean that you must recognize Self as the opposite of not-Self. Self has no duality. BLISS is beyond bliss and sorrow; it transcends both. Unconditioned Consciousness does not mean awareness as opposed to insensitivity. When you just spoke of "existence," you implied that there is a *state* of existence which is the opposite of nonexistence. And you spoke of this state in a way which would lead us to conclude that you consider such existence *desirable* and its opposite, nonexistence, *undesirable*. In other words, you are implying that you *want to be* and you *don't want not to be*. Is this not so?

Student (After a pause): Yes, I see what you mean.

RH: So, that being the case, I answer your question by telling you that, in Reality, *you do not exist* in the sense in which you are conceiving "existence" as the opposite of "nonexistence." Because you do not so exist in what you call "life," you do not so exist in what you think of as "death." But Self always IS. If you can recognize this "IS," then you always EXIST. Once you Know that you EXIST, you are no longer troubled with the illusions of life and death. You Understand life and death as waves that take their forms from the ocean but can never be apart from the ocean, from SELF.

Student: Would it be correct, then, to say that "everything exists in Self"?

RH: Nothing exists *in* Self. There is nothing apart from Self that exists *within* it and that can go *out* from it. Self IS. Do the rays of the sun exist *in* the sun? No, the rays *are* the sun. The nature of the ordinary mind is to divide, split, separate, dissect, diversify, make many of the ONE, present the many as *apart* from the ONE and, ultimately, have the many entirely obscure the ONE. In this way, the parts become "real" and the ONE is concealed. But regardless of how the rays of the sun are examined, analyzed, broken into a spectrum, or transformed into energy, they remain the sun—not an "aspect" of the sun or a "part" of the sun or something that is emanating "from" the sun, but the *sun itself*. In the same way, regardless of how ordinary mind examines, analyzes, divides, and transforms in order to depict the phenomenal world to you in a particular way, ALL IS SELF.

Student: Why do we have such illusions of seeing the ONE as many? Where do they come from?

RH: They do not "come" and they do not "go." Imagine that you are taking a walk and you mistake a rope that is lying across the road, for a snake. You are startled and you react: you run away, or you get a stick to beat it, or whatever. But all your reactions have no basis; they are the result of faulty perception, of mistaking the rope for a snake. When at last you see that the snake is really a rope, do you ask, "Where has the snake gone to?" No. You know there has been no snake at all. You relax and have no further reactions to the illusory snake. So, the rope is always the rope even when there is the illusion that it is a snake. Self is always Self even when it is imagined in other forms. And all your reactions to these imagined forms are without basis.

Student: So the objective of our practice is to understand these illusions?

RH: An illusion cannot be "understood." Either you see the snake or you see the rope; you cannot see both simultaneously. You will recall the "cube" *yantra* that we looked at the other day. If you recognize your true nature, Self, then ordinary mind, illusion, cannot arise. You will not inquire, "Where has ordinary mind gone?" You will Know there has been no ordinary mind.

Student: Wherever you turn these days you are ordered to "get involved." In view of what we have been discussing here, this directive to "get involved" seems pretty pointless.

RH: Well, society and the media are requesting that you direct your actions into particular areas. Do whatever you must do. But Know that all actions performed from the center, from Self, are actionless. All actions performed with the sense of "*I* am doing this," generate karma.

Student: You say to "do whatever we must." But *must* we do anything?"

RH: Whatever you do is what you must do. You may believe that you plan, choose, and direct your actions, but in Reality there is never "something to be done" and one who "does" it. There is only spontaneous action without a "doer." Recognize that you are not the "doer."

Another Student: For the past several days I've been listening very carefully to all that has been said and this is the first time I'm speaking out—because I think I have something meaningful to add. I would like to tell the group that my personal experiences have been such that I can confirm, without doubt, the truth of what you have been teaching. I think it's remarkable how close you are able to bring us to God-consciousness through verbal means. When I am experiencing what you have referred to as "Self-awareness," it completely defies any type of verbal description. You simply cannot talk about it; I wouldn't even attempt to do so. So I'm really astonished that just through listening to you, this experience of Self has become very vivid to me on several occasions during the past few meetings. When I left yesterday's session I remembered something that might interest the group. I once went with several friends to hunt for a particular wild flower called a "shooting star." We went to an area where we were told we would find it and walked through a number of fields for about an hour looking for it. Then we became tired and sat down to rest in one particular field. While I was sitting there I began to look closely at the ground just beneath my legs and suddenly I saw a shooting star. I pointed it out to my friends and we began to look a little beyond where we were sitting and we saw that there were more shooting stars. Then we stood up and began to walk around and we saw that the entire field—which was very large—was completely covered with shooting stars. Imagine! We had walked through that same field a few minutes earlier and hadn't seen one shooting star; now we saw that the ground was covered with them. Somehow, they had been obscured from our view, but once we saw the first one we realized that this was an entire field of shooting stars. As a matter of fact, I couldn't see anything in this field *but* shooting stars. I'm telling you this story because I realized that this was just the way in which I first experienced what I call "God-consciousness." I caught just the tiniest glimpse of this consciousness and then I suddenly saw it everywhere, in everything. There was nothing that was *not* this consciousness.

RH: Thank you for telling us. That's a most illuminating analogy. Extremely graphic.

(Pause)

Whereas at one point you are looking for Self, you later realize that there is no way you can escape Self.

Student: Whenever I am able to move myself into what you have referred to as the "center," the experience seems to be the same. First, I perceive just the smallest ray of light, and almost immediately thereafter everything is totally illuminated and *I* am the center from which the radiation is emanating.

I must also say that this experience is becoming more frequent. I'm still unable to bring it on at will; it comes of its own accord, but it comes more frequently. I'm anxious to seriously apply some of the techniques I've learned here. . . .Oh, I also want to confirm another thing you've told us. When I'm in the center it is utterly inconceivable that I've ever been anywhere *but* in the center.

Another Student (Addressing the first student): Do you have this consciousness only during meditation or at other times also?

First Student: Oh, yes. It's at all different times. I've even had it while sleeping.

Another Student (Addressing the first student): What brings you out of the center?

First Student: I don't know. As I said, I'm anxious to apply some of the things we've discussed here.

Another Student (Addressing RH): What brings her out of the center?

RH: She hasn't gone in and she hasn't come out—no more than you have. You are seeing the rope as a snake. Self neither "comes" nor "goes."

Another Student: She mentioned experiencing Self during sleep. How can you practice to do this?

RH: You are always Self, sleeping or waking. When you get into bed and close your eyes, observe your breathing. Fix your attention on your breathing and hold it there. Investigate that place from where the breath arises and to where it goes. There you will find the origin of the "I." Continue this investigation as you pass into the sleep state.

Student: Is the enlightened person *conscious* of Self during sleep?

RH: The enlightened person neither sleeps nor wakes. The ordinary man, identifying with a body, transfers this identity to the enlightened man and sees him as sleeping and waking, working and resting, growing old and dying. But the enlightened man, Self, does none of these.

Student: Do you "initiate" your serious students into your teachings?

RH: Initiation [*diksha*] is usually envisioned as a formal ritual conducted by the guru, during which the student may be touched, given a mantra, presented with a new name, and so forth. However, I concur with Ramana Maharshi's technique of initiation through "silence." In this sense, you were all initiated when we sat together in silent meditation.

Student: Is it true that at the time of initiation certain secret knowledge is passed to the student and an eternal relationship is then established between the disciple and the guru?

RH: There is no "secret" knowledge that is pertinent to Self-recognition. The function of the true guru is to push the student within and terminate the student's dependence upon him, in any form, as quickly as possible, not to create a protracted relationship, transmit "secret" knowledge, confer a new name, and so forth. There are teachers who consider these devices helpful. This is their prerogative. I do not discern that there is a point of demarcation where an initiation should occur. That is, I do not recognize that there is a time when a seeker is a novice, and that he eventually reaches a point where he is to be formally considered as having progressed to another stage, at which time he is ready to be "initiated." The seeker is *always* ripe to recognize his true nature; each time he turns his mind inward he is initiated. The seeker who believes that he needs to be initiated, and receive whatever it is that he fantasizes is necessary for his enlightenment, may forget the business at hand.

Student: Do you think that initiation is mostly a psychological thing? I mean, if the student believes something has been done by the guru to awaken or alter his consciousness, then perhaps it really happens.

RH: The external guru utilizes various devices to "push" the seeker inside. The internal guru pulls and guides from within. If ordinary mind convinces you that you require these external pushes, then you will seek various ways of being "pushed." I told you the other day that I know of many seekers who have wasted years of time, which might have been devoted to practice, in looking for a physical guru. Again, one wants to go to the beach by way of Chicago. You need only *turn* inward, but you go far and wide seeking various means by which you will be *pushed* inward. What is the sense of searching or waiting for gurus, initiations, secret knowledge, rites, and so forth? At some point these things *may* manifest externally for you. In the meantime, practice your Yoga; turn inward.

Another Student: You said that students have wasted years of time. But is such time really "wasted"?

RH: I use this word to impress upon the ordinary mind of the seeker that all "time" spent looking for fulfillment in an external world is unproductive. The search for a guru, initiation, and so forth is to be considered in the same context: this search perpetuates the duality of a self that is looking for Self. This is an instance in which you may think that because the desire and search are for instruction or enlightenment, they are noble and purposeful, as opposed to the desire for sense gratification, which you may characterize as "objectionable" or "unspiritual." But the truth is that *all* desire and *all* search proceed from the ordinary mind and are equally futile in Self-recognition. You ARE SELF NOW.

Another Student: You implied that you *do* initiate in "silence." What is the procedure?

RH: In our doctrine, turning the mind inward is initiation, regardless of where or when this occurs. I perform no rites to induct students into a sect or organization. I said that if you meditated with us in any of the morning sessions or in the manner we have suggested, by yourself, you have been initiated. In our private consultations a number of you have acknowledged the experience of this initiation, although you may not have designated it as such. Turning the mind inward is initiation, regardless of whether or not you have an experience that is dramatic, emotional, illuminating, elevating, energizing, or whatever.

Student: Is your physical presence necessary for this type of initiation?

RH: No. Those who practice Yoga seriously by using my books and recordings, or through the instruction I offer on my television programs, know of my presence. Those of you who are here will always know that my presence is with you, if that is what you wish. But my presence is of small consequence in comparison with the presence of the one who guides you from within. Turn inward and you will contact *that* presence.

Student: My mind continues to raise doubts about whether I am practicing correctly.

RH: Yes, the illusion "doubts" the illusion. Find the *source* of the doubts; find the one who is doubting. There is no point in removing one doubt at a time because for each one that is removed, ten will take its place. One must go directly to the source. Doubts are extinguished when you find that the doubter is nonexistent.

Student: I've been meditating regularly and seriously for about a year. The thing that seems to affect me most is to see or hear about people suffering. If I am attempting to prevent my mind from flowing outward and I happen to observe an incident in which someone is hurt or suffering, I cannot restrain it. I become involved in his or her suffering.

RH: *Who* sees the suffering? You believe that the suffering

---

is apart from you, in a subject-object relationship. Find out about your own reality and then you will know if the suffering is real. You say that you cannot keep your mind inward when you observe suffering. But if your mind was turned within you would not "see" the suffering.

Student: Do you close your eyes to suffering?

RH: No, just the contrary. You *open* your eyes and understand the nature of suffering. Now you suffer because your eyes are *closed*. You experience suffering and project that suffering into an external world. If you wish to terminate suffering, find out *who* it is that suffers; trace suffering to the place whence it arises.

Student: For most of my life I have worshiped God in the traditional way, through prayer, supplication, petition, and so on. Now I am confused as to whether I should abandon this worship and simply meditate according to what I have learned here.

RH: There is no need to abandon worship. When you are at a certain level of understanding you see yourself as inferior to One whom you conceive as superior; you designate the superior One as "God" and proceed to worship Him in a subject-object relationship. Then there comes a point when God manifests as the inner guide and draws the ego, the I, the self, inward. At this point the inferior-superior, subject-object relationship ceases and the self recognizes that its nature is—and always has been—Self. This progression is the natural course of events and there need be no dichotomy or confusion. When the time comes, you will recognize that what you have been worshiping is your own true nature.

Another Student: You said before that you do not acknowledge a stage of readiness or ripeness for enlightenment. Now you say that there is such a time.

RH: What I have just outlined *appears as a progression* to the ordinary mind of the seeker. Once abiding in Self, he recognizes that this progression, this stepwise evolution, this gradual development, has been a dream of the self. Understand that Self has no gradations; you cannot *evolve* into Self. You ARE SELF.

Another Student: So, one may *worship*, as an alternative to other methods?

RH: One may surrender the self totally to the object of worship. This self-surrender [Bhakti Yoga] is the anticipation of self merging with Self. But remember that this surrender is absolute and complete. You take no further responsibility for your life and there is no further intervention of the ego. You "lose your life."

Student: But if there is no intervention of the ego, that is already the ultimate state. Can this complete surrender be accomplished so immediately?

RH: The student who undertakes to practice self-surrender develops the awareness to detect when the ego is manifesting. Each time he senses that he is in the clutches of the ego, that the "I" is once again directing his activities in an attempt to satisfy its incessant desires, he implements the self-surrender technique: he relinquishes the self, the unreal, to the object of his worship, to his conception of the Supreme. In this way, the hold of the ego is weakened and it reappears less and less.

Student: Can you tell me which path is the right one for me?

RH: Whichever is the easiest for you; whichever you are drawn to. All paths mingle and become one path. They are like tributaries of a river: whichever you follow eventually mixes with the others, and all return, as one river, to the source.

Student: If you join a particular sect or decide to follow the teachings of a particular guru and eventually you feel that you are not making progress or that that guru is not the right one for you, should you change the sect or seek another guru?

RH: Consult the guru within. Make yourself receptive to him and you will be guided.

Another Student: How do you do that?

RH: Turn inward and listen. He is always instructing. You said that you pray and worship. Don't you know that *he* is the one to whom you are praying?

Student: I see. I must reflect on this. . . . I mentioned before that I was now uncertain about prayer and worship. I think that part of this uncertainty stems from someone associated with my church. When I happened to mention to him that I was interested in Yoga, he told me that the practice of Yoga can be dangerous.

RH: What is the danger?

Student: He didn't specify.

RH: But he has experienced this danger?

Student: I don't know. Actually, I don't think he knows very much about Yoga.

RH: And yet he was able to influence you with such a vague, uninformed statement?

(The student did not reply.)

RH: If one has apprehension regarding the practice, it is best to back off. Yoga does not proselytize and seeks no "converts."

Student: I guess I just have too many doubts.

RH: No, you probably have too few. If and when you have *many* doubts, you may recognize that Yoga represents the resolution of these doubts and the insecurity and suffering which they generate. Then there will be no question about your attraction to Yoga.

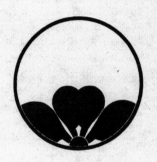

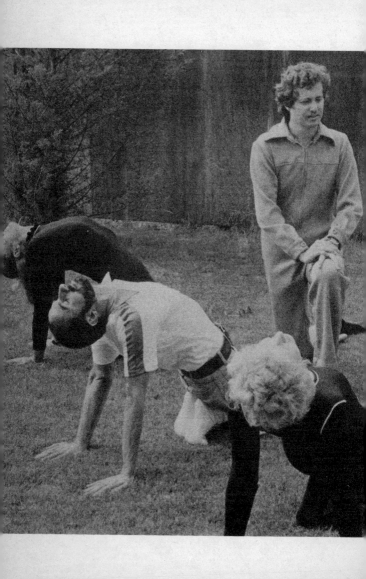

6th day

Student: I find myself being very critical of people. I believe that this is my worst habit. I am continually criticizing, but actually I don't want to be doing so. Can you give me any suggestion?

RH: All habits, traits of personality, and behaviorial patterns that are considered both favorable and unfavorable, constructive and destructive, proceed from one source. What is the advantage of examining and attempting to eliminate one bad habit at a time? There is no end to bad habits; you will never finish with them because the entity that is examining the habits and evaluating them as "bad" is the same entity that is creating them! Rather, seek the *source* of their emanation. When the projector in the movie house is turned off, all of the good and bad action that has been occurring on the screen, and all the actors who are portraying good and bad roles disappear instantaneously. The bad ones don't disappear first, or disappear one by one, or disappear a little bit at a time. When the medium through which the illusion is manifesting (the projector) is turned off, the entire illusion is gone all at once. Find your projector and put an end to *all* your illusions with one stroke.

Another Student: I notice that sometimes you say *"seek* the source" and at other times *"find* the source." Are these two different things?

RH: They are the same. We undertake to "seek" so that we can "find." But through practice you will understand that what appears to be the means—the seeking—is actually the goal. In the course of your practice, the "seeking" is transformed into the "finding." Always be aware that there is nothing to be attained or acquired in this practice. You "get" nothing. If there was something to acquire, something that you do not now have and have never had, it would be temporal, transient, elusive, vaporous, and not worth acquiring. It is more accurate to describe Yoga as a practice which *uncovers what appears to be obscured.*

Another Student: I want to ask you about renunciation. You say to "surrender self." Along with this surrender, is it not a very meaningful act to surrender your possessions, to offer them to God? In order to become a member of certain sects in both the East and the West, it is necessary to give up all possessions and live in poverty. I would like to hear your comments on this.

RH: We must understand the real meaning of "surrender." Imagine that there is a man who, while attending services in a church, finds a twenty-dollar bill on the floor which he knows has fallen from the collection plate. At a later time he "donates" this same bill to the same church as a gesture of his charity. Now, the bill was not his to take, he did not own it while it was in his possession, and therefore it was not his to "donate" as an act of charity. So it is with your possessions. They are not yours to "own" and therefore cannot be "surrendered" or donated as a gesture of your renunciation. For those who are of a particular nature and at a certain level of understanding, the act of abandoning their possessions and living in physical poverty is chosen as an overt way to be continually reminded of the ultimate condition: nothing is truly "owned" and God is to be totally relied upon to fulfill all one's needs. So, abandon or do not abandon your possessions, as you will. True asceticism lies in Knowing that nothing can ever be yours to give or take. True renunciation is the renunciation of all that is of the not-Self: ego, I, self, ordinary mind.

Another Student: Jesus said, "It is easier for a camel to go through the eye of a needle than for a rich man to enter the kingdom of heaven."

RH: Of course. If a man thinks of himself as wealthy, he must protect what he believes to be his wealth, and his attachment to and identification with his possessions precludes his becoming free of them and recognizing his true nature. But an enlightened King Solomon or King Asoka can exist as liberated beings despite their enormous wealth. What you "own" is of no consequence. How you regard what you own is everything.

Student: I wonder if I might ask you to clarify a few points about meditation while practicing Hatha Yoga. I know you refer to this as "active meditation" and I'd like to hear exactly what this means.

RH: The instructors in your Hatha classes here have been presenting information along these lines—especially in the advanced classes—but perhaps I can add a few words that will prove helpful.

I use the words *active* and *passive*, in the context of meditation, only in the physical sense: either you are moving and acting or you are stationary and sitting in the meditative pose. In the actual technique, that is, in the inward turning of the mind, there is no distinction as to active or passive. Because a series of physical movements comprise most of the asanas, fixing the

---

mind and holding it steady while performing these asanas is designated "active" meditation.

The method of active meditation consists of two techniques. First, the consciousness is firmly fixed on the movements. You become acutely aware of what parts of the body are involved in the asana; you *feel* all that is involved. During the static "hold" of the asana you direct the consciousness to that area which is being emphasized or stressed. In this way, the mind is one-pointed and is prevented from wandering. From the moment you begin your practice session, the attention is totally confined to the movements. This restraint of the mind, this turning inward of the consciousness is not only effective meditation but definitely increases the physical benefits of the practice.

The second technique of active meditation during Hatha Yoga practice is that of *visualization*. Here, the consciousness is occupied with a particular *yantra* [geometrical figure] while you are in the static position of a particular asana. These yantras are depicted in the charts that are displayed in our advanced classes here and are also reproduced in my *8 Steps to Health and Peace* book.

An extremely valuable aspect of "active" meditation is that learning to fix and hold the consciousness while moving in the asanas enables you to extend this technique more and more into the activities of your everyday life. All that you do begins to assume the form of active meditation.

Student: And following the Hatha Yoga session, do you do the "passive" meditation?

RH: Yes. I suggest that procedure.

Student: Could I continue to meditate on one of the yantras that I used in the Hatha practice?

RH: Yes, or any one of several techniques that I have suggested and that you are experimenting with in our morning meditation classes. Those who are attracted to the inquiry method—"Who Am I?"—should utilize that. The principal objective for the beginning meditator is to retract the senses and the mind from the external world, fix the attention on whatever you have selected as the object for concentration or meditation, and hold it there with as little fluctuation as possible until fatigue sets in. Try to be aware of the distinction between fatigue and restlessness. Fatigue manifests as weariness or exhaustion and indicates that your practice session should be terminated. Restlessness is the itch of the mind to turn back into the external world; from this it should be gently restrained. The importance of this restraint might be pointed up if you will imagine that you have a painful sore which is causing you severe discomfort. Rather than apply a soothing salve to protect the sore from further irritation, so that it may heal, you elect to take a pointed instrument and jab it, at regular intervals, into this sore. Such a course of action would be considered sheer madness. But consider your situation in maya. You find yourself in a condition—which you define as "living"—that is causing you severe and continual pain. Rather than recognize your true nature, which would terminate your pain, you perpetuate this suffering—you regularly jab the wound—by permitting your ordinary mind to flow outward, to conceptualize without restraint. Turning the mind inward is like applying the salve; holding the mind inward is like the protection which effects healing.

Another Student: If you know you are dying, what should you attempt to envision at the moment of death?

RH: Find out if you are now "alive" before you concern yourself with "death."

Student: Would you elaborate on that?

RH: You have identified yourself with a body. You know that the body dies and so you think that you also die. But your true nature, Self, is not born and does not die. Recognize your true nature.

Student: The *Tibetan Book of the Dead* and certain other esoteric treatises present directions for guiding one through the after-death experience.

RH: If you are lending reality to life and death, and distinguishing between them, then it is incumbent upon you to put forth whatever efforts are necessary while you are "alive" to recognize your true nature.

Student: But what if you cannot accomplish it in this lifetime?

RH: Ask yourself *who* it is that believes there is something to be "accomplished" and *who* it is that thinks about "this lifetime." If you find the "I," you will understand that there is nothing to be accomplished. Then, the illusion of "lifetimes" and "deathtimes" will dissolve. When the Yogic texts describe the liberated man as having "conquered death," it is this dissolution of self that is indicated.

Student: I have been attracted to the "Who Am I?" meditation since first reading about it in your *Meditation* book [*Guide to Yoga Meditation*] several years ago. But when I attempt it I seem to tire quickly—I become restless and give it up after a few minutes. But then, a few days later, I am again drawn to it, and the same thing happens.

RH: The fact that you are continually attracted to this inquiry should be encouraging. Rather than making spasmodic attempts, which you indicate are a few days or weeks apart, you should practice regularly each day—perhaps twice each day. In this way your restlessness, which is the itch of the ordinary mind to run rampant and unconstrained in its fantasies, will decrease. You cannot train a wild animal without regular training sessions. The same is true of the ordinary mind. Through persistence you will come to recognize the nature of the adventure on which you have embarked in undertaking Yoga practice and meditation. When this recognition occurs, nothing will prevent you from regular meditation because now the magnetic direction is reversed: the magnetism of Self, pulling you inward, overpowers the tendencies [*vasanas*] of ordinary mind to pull you outward into its illusions.

Student: So, as long as I am attracted to this method I should continue with it and not attempt something different?

RH: As I have repeatedly said: one should trust and follow one's intuition, one's attraction. The guru within guides, and for the beginner this guidance manifests as "attraction."

Student: It seems virtually impossible for me to suppress my desires and passions. It seems to require the type of strength that I'm just not able to muster.

RH: Nothing has been said about "suppressing" passions. That is a futile approach. What good is suppression, which, at best, can only be fleeting? Suppressed desires soon arise again. I have instructed you not to "suppress," but to determine the *source* of your desires. To *whom* do these desires come and from *where* do they arise? Only in understanding the *nature* of desires can you prevent them from consuming you.

Student: Are the thoughts of certain acts, such as lust and violence, as harmful as the act themselves?

RH: You believe that these thoughts are *your* thoughts, but they are actually the inventions of the computer, of ordinary mind. They emanate from ordinary mind and circulate through the minds of all ordinary men and women. Everyone entertains these thoughts, as well as thoughts—in one form or another—about everything else in the world of phenomena. You may believe that your thoughts are "hidden" from others, that no other person thinks or perceives what *you* are thinking. But that is an aspect of the ordinary mind's illusion. Every person has these same thoughts who has not discerned the nature of ordinary mind. Not all people have the same ordinary-mind thoughts simultaneously, but these thoughts are continually circulating like an electrical current making a circuit; sooner or later they all pass through what you believe to be *your* mind. You mentioned "violence and lust." These thoughts circulate through everyone and, according to his or her makeup, evoke varying reactions. But all who have not recognized their true nature are vulnerable to these thoughts—as well as to all other thoughts.

You are aware of a thought and you say, "I am thinking about . . ." and this thought occupies your attention, perhaps for a moment, perhaps for many years. But for however long it remains, you believe it to be *your* thought. Does the current belong to the light bulb? No, it is part of a circuit passing through the bulb, and, depending upon the type of circuit it may light the bulb for only an instant or for a lengthy interval. But we know that the current can be terminated entirely, at any time, by turning off the switch.

Student: But one person can have a violent thought and contain it—that is, not react overtly—and another person has the same thought and runs amok with a hatchet.

RH: Precisely. Also, the same person may react differently at different times to the identical thought. So, rather than be concerned as to the distinction between thought and action, it is best to find the place from *where* the thoughts arise, to find the it that turns the current on and off. Then you will understand that you neither think nor act. *It is not your thought*; consequently, you cannot react to it in any way. *Your* thoughts and *your* actions are illusions.

Another Student: How can these thoughts arise and circulate through mankind if they are illusory?

RH: Illusion is the nature of ordinary mind and the state of maya, which it invents and sustains. It's the Emperor's New Clothes syndrome. Imagine a crowded bus in which someone with a perverted sense of humor wants to play a practical joke. He screams, "Fire! Fire!" and begins to run toward the exit. His false panic spreads instantaneously and all stampede toward the exit. But the wise man will say, "Hold your places. *Where* is the fire?" In the same way, before you are stampeded by your desires into seeking fulfillment in an illusory world, determine from *where* these desires and thoughts are arising. Find out *who* is stampeding you.

RH: Some of you have indicated that you can intellectually grasp the idea that the phenomenal world is an illusion—in the sense that it is a projection of ordinary mind—but that you are unable to discern how the one who is *seeing* the illusion—the "I"—is also an illusion. Perhaps an illustration will prove helpful.

Have you ever seen a movie in which two of the actors in this movie go into a theater and also watch a movie? And in the movie you are watching, one of the actors begins to speak to the other about the movie *they* are watching. They discuss this movie and react to what is taking place. But you know that the actors who are watching and talking about the movie are also *in* the movie. So, *you* know that what the actors are seeing in the movie *they* are watching is an illusion, and you know that the actors themselves, the ones who are witnessing the action, are also illusory. In the same way, that which you see in the world is illusory, like the movie that is being watched by the actors, and the one who is seeing the illusion—the one you refer to as "I"—is also an illusion, like the actors who are watching the movie. Both that which is seen and the ones who are seeing are illusory.

The only reality in the whole business is the screen upon which all of this is transpiring. While the movie—the illusion—is playing, you are hypnotized by the action, and you are oblivious to the screen even though you could see nothing without it. When the movie has ended, and the projector is turned off and the house lights are turned on, the screen remains unchanged. But now its reality is quite apparent because there is nothing to distract you from seeing it. In a similar way, *you* are the screen, Self, unchanging, regardless of whether or not the illusions of "that which is seen" and "he who sees" appear upon it.

(There was an interval of silence while the group considered these remarks.)

Student: In the example you've just given, there is still the one in the real theater who knows that he's watching an illusion within an illusion.

RH: That one, who is sitting in what you call the "real" theater *is also within a movie*, and the one who *sees* him sitting in the "real" theater is also within a movie, and so on forever. The illusion is infinite; it is like placing two mirrors face to face and then attempting to determine which of the multiple reflections are real and which are illusions. Obviously, they are *all* reflections, and hence they are all unreal. In the same way, each of your "I's" that attempts to stand back and objectify another "I" is an illusion. Both the subject and the object are unreal. That which is seen and the one who is seeing are mirages.

Student: But can the original two mirrors that have been placed face to face be considered real?

RH: For the purpose of this illustration, we may say that the mirrors are real but not the reflections that appear in them, just as we may say that the screen is real but not the illusions that appear upon it. Your true nature can be conceived as approximating the mirror and the screen, upon which images appear but have no reality and cannot affect them. Understand, however, that these examples are given only for the purpose of accommodating ordinary mind, accomodating it so that we may expose its nature. Self-consciousness recognizes no mirrors or screens, no projections, no reflections, and no illusions. SELF IS. "I AM," said the Lord.

Student: The Hindus designate three states of existence: waking, dreaming and dreamless sleep. Do you acknowledge that there are such states and that one is more important than the others?

RH: You say "three states of existence." EXISTENCE—which transcends existence and nonexistence—is

---

synonymous with SELF. There is nothing of Self that is of more consequence than something else; Self is All in All. You have only one "state": *sat-chit-ananda*, Existence-Knowledge-Bliss.

Student: But it seems that we can only practice Yoga in the waking state. For those of us who have not realized the ultimate objective, the waking state would be the most important.

RH: There is no "ultimate objective" to realize. You have only to give up the unreal which you are mistaking for the real. When construction workers prepare the foundation for a building, they excavate the earth and are left with a hole. They do not "make" a hole. The hole is the natural consequence of the earth being removed. Self is the natural consequence of removing the not-Self.

Regarding your observation about the "waking" state: if you have not recognized that your true nature is Yoga, meditation, and that you do not sleep or wake but only meditate, then you can practice to understand this even during sleep. I have already described the technique of observing the breath when retiring for the night.

Another Student: I wanted to comment on this technique the other day but didn't have the opportunity. You told us about it last year and I've been attempting to apply it but I haven't really succeeded. I can do it for a short time, but then my mind wanders before the moment I actually do fall asleep and then I think I just dream . . . but I'm pretty sure I don't meditate.

RH: Then do whatever you can while you're awake. Gradually, sufficient strength will be gained so that you can extend the practice into sleep.

Another Student: Are dreams of any value? There are those who believe that dreams can reveal important things hidden in our subconscious.

RH: You are saying that illusions can "reveal" illusions about your illusions. If you mistake fantasy for Reality, then there will be no end of dreams, revelations, and things that are "hidden." Once you recognize Self you will understand that nothing is hidden, that everything has already been revealed, and that your existence in maya, whether awake or asleep, is a "dream" of the ordinary mind.

Another Student: Since I was here last year I've been meditating. There are times when I can actually feel myself functioning in this illusory state. But when I attempt to examine it, it slips away. You can't get a handle on it.

RH: Of course; it's the ultimate illusion. Ordinary mind cannot withstand closeup scrutiny. So, although it may indulge you in peripheral examination of itself by itself—to convince you that it is fair and objective—it will create every possible obstacle to prevent the ultimate inquiry: *finding its source*. The magician may open the door of his illusion box to show there is nothing inside when the audience is at a safe distance. But does he invite the audience backstage or into his dressing room before the performance so that they can observe him setting up the show?

You will recall the fall of a recent national administration. It knew it could not prevail if the investigation was dedicated and thorough. So its leader told us that *he* had investigated and had taken the proper action to correct the situation. In other words, the conspirators had investigated the conspiracy in the same way that ordinary mind would have you accept that it has investigated itself and done whatever is necessary to prevent further deceptions from arising. But when the investigators refused to accept this reassurance and, in continuing their investigation, began to home in on the crux of the matter, the conspirators initiated many devices to forestall further inquiry. Delays, the Fifth Amendment, "executive privilege" were all invoked. But the investigators persevered and, in the end, the conspiracy could not withstand the exposure. In the same way, *you* must persevere in your investigation.

You commented that you were having trouble examining the illusory state. Remember that "examining the illusion" is like ordinary mind investigating itself, the conspirators investigating the conspiracy. Abandon any examination of the illusion. *Find that place from where the illusion arises.* Time and again the ordinary mind will inform you that the investigation has been concluded and that it has implemented whatever is necessary to rectify the illusory condition. But this is all part of the conspiracy. Persist in your inquiries, *"Who Am I?"* and *"Where Am I?"* until the ordinary mind and its manifold inventions are recognized as phantoms. Whenever ordinary mind detects that you are approaching this objective, it will, for self-preservation, pull out all the stops: delays, diversions, distractions, executive privilege. *Persist in turning it inward.*

Student: I've been applying what I have learned here in answering a riddle and I'd like to know if my conclusion corresponds with what you would answer. It's the riddle of the tree falling in the forest: if no one is there to hear it fall, does it make a sound?

RH: You see how the ordinary mind would suck us in?
(Pause)
Let me ask you this: Do you still beat your wife?
(Laughter)
Well, let us give you the benefit of the doubt and assume that you do not now and never have beaten your wife. So, you would reply, "The question is irrelevant. You are basing your question on the assumption that I formerly beat my wife. You should have asked me if I had *ever* beaten her, and if I had said, 'Yes,' *then* you could have asked me if I *still* beat her." In the same way, you base your "tree" riddle on the assumption that there is a noise that *can* or *cannot* be heard. You should first inquire if anyone has *ever* heard the sound of a tree falling. Is there actually one who hears [subject] and a sound that is heard [object]? You see how ordinary mind divides itself into subject and object and plays one against the other? It would have us believe

that there is a question created by *external* conditions [in this case, about the noise of a falling tree] which can be answered by the *internal* mind. *But all the time the ordinary mind is both question and answer, both subject and object!* There is neither a tree which falls nor one to hear it fall.

Student: Yes, I see. . . .It is not what I would have answered.

Another Student: So, if I am not present to observe or hear any phenomenon, that phenomenon does not occur?

RH: *Nothing* "occurs." The mind, flowing outward, gives rise to an "I" or to many "I's" that observe and react to phenomena. The mind, turned inward, merges with its source, Self, from which no such phenomena can arise.

Student: Let me press this further. I am now here, but at my home, which is in Indianapolis, I am reasonably sure that certain things are happening. My children are attending school and my husband is at work. Although I am imagining that this is the case, I am almost certain that when I arrive back home I will find that these things have occurred. My point is that I do not need to be at home to know that certain things are occurring, no more than I need to be in the forest to know that a falling tree creates a sound.

RH: The events that you imagine are occurring at your home have no more reality than the events you are observing here. All these events are proceeding from ordinary mind. Ordinary mind evaluates some things as "real" because the senses are directly involved—such as our speaking together here—and some things as "imagined" because images are conjured up independently of the senses. But *all* imaginings, together with all interpretations of phenomena by the senses, are the illusions of ordinary mind. Therefore, nothing in maya is more "real" than anything else. So, I reiterate: rather than endless speculation as to whether or not there is a noise, determine the origin of the one who is concerned about the noise.

Student: What do you think of the Women's Liberation Movement? I am actively involved in it.

RH: All women and men who have not recognized their true natures are in bondage. All are liberated as Self.

Another Student: Most religious and philosophical organizations attempt to get involved in the activities of their communities. Should Yogis do the same?

RH: Those who practice Yoga according to the pure doctrine do not consider themselves members of any organization. They have no desire to promote themselves as benefactors. Each does as it comes to her to do. If she offers her services to the community, she does so without the sense of doership and certainly does not announce that her help or services are associated with her Yoga practice. She seeks no recognition from the community or from society. Work and service are performed because it comes to one to do so, never for reward or recognition.

Student: How do you account for the fact that those who we know to be Self-realized beings, the great saints and so forth, seem to offer instruction that is frequently different and even in conflict?

RH: Not only does it appear that these teachings differ among the teachers, but that the same teacher offers different instruction to the same disciples at different times! One must understand that, since all such instruction proceeds from Self, there is no actual difference, but that each instructs according to the capacity for understanding among his students or of a particular student. This capacity is different among different peoples at different times and even a student who asks the identical question on a number of occasions may receive different responses—as the teacher perceives that the capacity of this student has increased.

Another Student: When you speak to us as a group, how do you determine the capacity for understanding of the group?

RH: In my general lectures I present the pure teachings as I perceive them, without regard to individual capacity. In *these* meetings, and in our private consultations, the teachings are modified or rephrased according to my perception of the student's level of understanding.

Student: I think this is a diplomatic way of telling us that some of us are not very bright.
  (Laughter)

RH: Not at all! Rephrasing or modification does not in any way alter the Truth of the teachings. They are simply presented in a different form. Many different objects may be made from gold, but the gold does not diminish in value by appearing in one form rather than another. See beyond the form and you find the substance. See beyond the form of the teachings and you find Self.

Another Student: How can one increase one's capacity for understanding?

RH: Through practice [*sadhana*]. Through Yoga and meditation. In Truth, capacity is not increased; rather, the student divests himself of the unreal, of the veils that obscure Self. In this way, it *appears* that capacity increases.

Another Student: How do you determine the level of understanding of your television viewers?

RH: That is a different matter. When one is instructing what are primarily *techniques* to several million people who may be totally unfamiliar with such techniques, it is necessary to present them in a modified form. This is the manner in which I instruct the Hatha Yoga asanas, pranayama, and meditation in the television series.

Student: I suppose you know that many of your viewers reach a point where they become very serious and want to go further, but they don't have access to a competent teacher and they don't know how to proceed.

RH: All who are practicing seriously will find the necessary guidance.

Student: I remember reading that the Buddhists believe the world does not exist. Am I correct in saying that you believe the world exists, but is unreal? And if this is your view, how do you reconcile it with the Buddhist view?

RH: In the East there are three basic views of phenomena. First, there is the view that acknowledges the existence of the world and that a man may seek his salvation in the world. The second view is that the world exists but is unreal in the sense that a mirage exists but is an illusion. The third view is that nothing, including the world and all phenomena, exists in any sense whatsoever. In our doctrine, there is no disparity among these three views; they form a natural progression in this way: a man begins to seek salvation, enlightenment, God, or whatever you wish to call it. Because the world appears real to him, he has no alternative but to seek his salvation in the world. Even if he conceives of God in the abstract—as a spirit, or as an entity abiding in an "unseen" region—he still seeks Him in and through the phenomenal world. Eventually, in the natural course of seeking, his consciousness is refined. He then continues to perceive the phenomenal world, but conceives that it is not external and apart from him; it appears to be manifesting *through* him. So, at this point he regards the world as illusory, as being projected from or through himself, but he still regards himself, the one who is observing the illusory world, as real. Ultimately, this second view evolves into the third: here, the self merges with Self and nothing of a phenomenal nature exists. There is no longer "view" or "nonview," "existence" or "nonexistence," but only EXISTENCE, only ONENESS.

These views may evolve into one another during the course of many lifetimes or within one lifetime. Such things are dependent on one's previous practice. The student must always be aware that his attraction to

Yoga and related practices is the consequence of previous study and practice, and that he is now ready to achieve the reintegrated state. Therefore, very serious practice becomes the major business of his life because it represents the expedient for terminating rebirth. However, let me reiterate that "views," "progressions," "stages," "reintegration," and so forth are all concepts of ordinary mind. *You are always Self and could never be otherwise.*

Student: About these "three views of existence": in the ultimate state, where all phenomena cease to exist, does one still function in the world—even though it is an illusory world—without difficulty? Does he see everything and react to everything?

RH: We have spoken of this a number of times. But since this is our final meeting of the series, now may be an appropriate time to reiterate some of the points that are pertinent to your question.

First, you see how tenaciously the ordinary mind holds on? The concern reflected by your question is that of "functioning" in the world. This is all-important to you. You still believe that your happiness and fulfillment are somehow dependent on continuing to function in the world. Until now, your frustration, exasperation, torment, despair, and all those things that have brought you to Yoga have endured precisely because you *have* "functioned in the world." Now we are pointing to the key which will unlock your cell and you are wondering if you aren't really better off in jail after all!

Next, your question implies that you want a description of the enlightened condition, but this is none other than your *true* state. The prisoner is asking what the outside world is like, so that he can decide whether or not he wishes to leave the jail. He's afraid that he may not be able to handle all that freedom. But is it his natural condition to be in jail or to be free?

The liberated man [*jnani*] sees nothing but Self, or rather IS nothing but Self. If he goes to the forest and lives there, then that is what he does. But if he remains in the city and crosses the street, do you think he will fail to see the automobiles approaching? that he is crossing the street in some sort of stupefied condition or hypnotic trance? Attempting to maintain its dominant position, ordinary mind fantasizes about the nature of Self-consciousness and may depict it as a condition of indifference, ineptitude, stupefaction, hypnosis, or whatever else will perpetuate your doubts and prevent you from recognizing Self. But ordinary mind can Know nothing of Self; the most it can do is speculate. Self emerges only when ordinary mind subsides. The moment you step out of the cell, you understand that you have never been in jail!

Another Student: Cannot things that we perceive in the world, such as great art and music, assist us in knowing Self?

RH: Everything is a path to Self. But what direction will the seeker who investigates external phenomena have to take? He will gradually come to recognize that the music and art, or whatever, exist only by virtue of his cognition of them. So then he will understand that art and music, as well as garbage and noise, lead to the one who sees and hears them. Thus, he must eventually turn inward.

Student: In Kundalini Yoga, the power which is to be aroused is at the base of the spine. But other systems place this power in different areas of the body, such as the heart and the head.

RH: Yes. It may be said that the basic *shakti* [force] has various locations. All are within the subtle body, not the physical body. One who becomes a student of a system should follow that system exclusively.

Ramana Maharshi taught that the "I" consciousness is in the heart-center, located at that point in the chest where one touches himself when he says, "I." He suggested that the student could direct his attention to

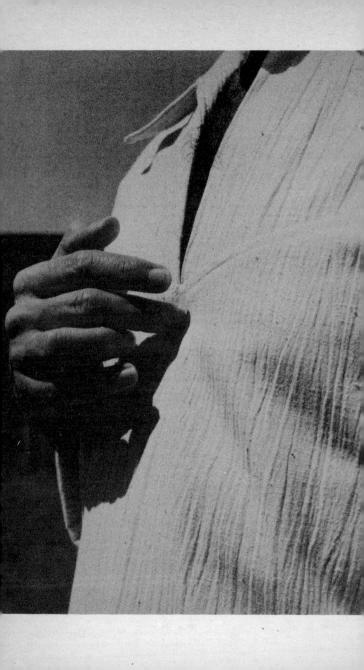

that area while he practiced the "Who Am I?" inquiry. You may wish to do the same.

Student: Is it advantageous to live a well-ordered, regulated life?

RH: You cannot "live a life" like a train travels on a track. You can only BE. All those whose minds flow outward are disordered and unregulated. When the mind is turned and held inward, you will have no concern as to order and disorder.

Student: But in terms of what will now help us to practice, aren't there guidelines for conducting one's life?

RH: I have discussed these "guidelines" in detail in my various Hatha Yoga books. For those of you who have attended these meetings, the principal guideline is this: whatever "structure" most facilitates your serious practice is the one to adopt.

Frequently, we look to others for examples on how to "conduct" our lives. But each person's path is individual and unique. Each has his own guide within. That is why I encourage students to look to themselves for instruction. Whenever I detect that a student is seeking to learn about his true nature from an external source—even if this source be the teachings of the saints or *avatars*—I attempt to redirect his efforts, to turn him into himself.

Another Student: I'm not sure what "avatar" means. Is it the same as "saint"?

RH: Vishnu is God in the form of the Preserver of the universe. Whenever a major alteration in the condition of man is necessary, an avatar, a direct manifestation of Vishnu or God, appears. If we think of the length of the Creation in biblical terms—that it extends from the paradisiacal condition before the fall of Adam, to a time when man shall be reinstated in that condition—we can speak of *ten* avatars who appear during this interval. The seventh of these is *Rama*, whose activities are recounted in the epic *Ramayana*; the eighth is *Krishna*, whose teachings are the subject of the *Bhagavad-Gita* [an excerpt from the epic *Mahabharata*]. The ninth avatar is one who effects a major transformation in the non-Hindu world; it is not clear from the Hindu scriptures whether this is Buddha or Christ—or perhaps both. The coming of the tenth avatar will mark the dissolution of sin, ignorance, etcetera, and the end of the present "dark" age [*Kali-yuga*]. Man will be reunited with Self. This tenth avatar of the Hindus is the one who is also awaited (by other names) by the major religions. This cosmology in no way influences the practice of the serious student. He is involved solely with the recognition of SELF, NOW.

Another Student: What is the principal difference between the actions of the enlightened man and the ordinary man? I mean, supposing they're both doing the same thing, what is the difference?

RH: The enlightened man has no sense of "doing" or of being the doer. Because his work is not generated by desire, he is liberated from the burden of action and the fruits of action.

Student: Will a person who is highly intelligent have a quicker and firmer grasp on these teachings? Does he understand them in a more immediate way than, say, one whose mind is not so developed? Even if we're talking about the ordinary mind, doesn't it help if it is knowledgeable in philosophy, the arts, methods of learning, and so forth?

RH: I think you are confusing scholastic aptitude with intelligence. I define the "intelligent person" as one who recognizes the illusory nature of his ordinary mind when he hears the doctrine and undertakes, without delay, the recommended practices. Any person may be of this "intelligent" nature. It is simply another way of saying that he is "ripe," that he has "ears to hear." Such intelligence has evolved from previous exposure to and application of the teachings; it has nothing to do with one's present occupation, environment, and so forth. The scriptures are replete with accounts of so-called "simple" persons who had no education but who, nonetheless, attained the highest spiritual status. Scholarship in no way furthers one's grasp of the doctrine of Self-consciousness; frequently, it acts as an impediment. No amount of exercise of the ordinary mind—in academic pursuits—can manifest Universal Mind.

[A student told the group about an organization which presents a method of self-development in a format of several weekend seminars, and asked Mr. Hittleman for his opinion. This is an organization which had been receiving much publicity in the media and the student's question was prompted by the fact that her husband was interested in attending the seminars.]

RH: One can pursue those things which attract him. However, I would say to those of you who may develop an interest in such organizations to determine if they are able to provide the serious seeker with the pure teachings or whether, through such appealing phrases as "develop your potential," they are really presenting formulas for "success." The quest for success is that of self-aggrandizement and cannot further one in the practice we have been discussing here. "What profit it a man if he should gain the whole world and lose his own soul?" If you are occupied with becoming "successful" you cannot devote the required attention to your practice. What the conspirators regard as "wealth" and "success" may come to you as the natural consequence of your karma. But to actively seek such things is to curtail your apprehension of the pure doctrine. This is the truth and there is no exception to it. So organizations—such the one you have mentioned—must be examined in that light: do they really furnish the means for Self-knowledge or do they obliquely offer to fulfill one's desire for self-aggrandizement? Once a determination has been made, you can proceed accordingly.

(Pause)

Many years ago, a man who attended a series of my lectures came to me at its conclusion and told me how much he had enjoyed and benefitted from having attended. Then he confided that he had been a member of a particular group for some years and that he had mastered a meditation technique which was developed by the instructor of the group. He invited me to come to his home and meditate with his group for the purpose of materializing a large amount of money. He told me that, without exception, each member of this group had become successful in business and in his or her personal life through this meditation technique. I explained to him that I did not participate in such activities; I further told him that the money and success that were "materialized" in this manner would impede his genuine apprehension of Truth. He thanked me for my teachings and went his way. The point I wish to make is that that gentleman sat through a series of twelve lectures and discussion groups in which I presented the same material as I have here, and he interpreted the program as one through which it might be possible to "materialize" money!

He is not alone in this interpretation. Millions of people regard prayer and meditation as a form of petition, as the means by which the desires and promises of ordinary mind may be fulfilled. Various teachers and organizations design their programs to appeal to those who harbor such desires. Some organizations make no bones about what they are offering: "Join our group and learn how God will grant what you want." Others make their appeal in a more subtle way, in the "develop your full potential" way. I am not suggesting that these organizations actively conspire to deceive. Their leaders and teachers have the identical need to fulfill desires. It may appear perfectly correct to them that, if they have found a way to fulfill desires, they should pass along the good news. They simply have not evolved to that point where the illusion and the futility of fulfilling any and all desires are understood. This is why I told you that it is most important for the Yoga instructor to explain the nature of Yoga in the early classes of the session, so that if the student is harboring illusions of fulfilling his desires through the Yoga practice, these illusions will be dispelled.

Other teachings that should be scrupulously avoided by the Yoga student are those characterized as "occult" or any which purport to develop "power." The desire to wield power and develop the ability to manipulate people and conditions, or to "control one's destiny," is, for many, irresistible. Certain organizations make their appeals directly to those who are desirous of achieving such things. So, if you ever detect that you are involved in such a study, I suggest you extricate yourself immediately. You will find it to be true that those who desire to control and manipulate others have little control of themselves; that, of course, is what makes them dangerous. This is why I also apprised you of the fact that you may very well reach a point in your practice where you realize that you *do* have access to "power," and that, at that point, you must observe this development with absolute detachment [*vairagya*]. Any utilization of such power will greatly circumscribe your progress.

Student: But according to what you said previously, regardless of whatever group or sect or organization one may become involved with, one is moving toward Self.

RH: Yes, but through indirection. *You* know the *direct* path. Recognize that you are Self, NOW. And remember that no one "moves toward Self." All ARE ALWAYS SELF.

Student: A meditation technique that you describe in one of your books is that of emptying the mind, thinking of nothing, having no thoughts. Do you recommend this technique for those of us who are here and who have heard you describe the "Who Am I?" method?

RH: Emptying the mind is a helpful technique for the beginner. As with *Observation of the Breath* and *Pranayama*, it aids in withdrawing the senses, quieting the mind, and preparing the mind to turn inward. But you must utilize it only in this context. Quieting the mind, "suspending" the thoughts, is only preparatory. If you stop here, the thoughts will just rise again. So, once you have developed some facility in withdrawal, focus the attention fully on the "Who Am I?" inquiry, or whatever is the seed, the object, of your meditation.

Student: It seems to me that fixing the attention on an object is more effective in preventing distracting thoughts than attempting to first empty the mind.

RH: This may be the case. It is a matter which must be left to each individual. Experiment and you will soon find which is the easiest for you.

Student: And the easiest is the best?

RH: Yes. It is your way.

Student: Is it possible for me to develop my own techniques—those which I may find easier than any of the traditional methods?

RH: It's possible, but it may require a lengthy period for these to evolve. The methods I have suggested are those that have been tested for many centuries and found to be effective. Also, I believe that both the number and diversity of the methods in which we have instructed you here have a sufficiently universal appeal so that each of you will be attracted to one or more of them. You will find that you cannot so readily develop an effective technique that is not included in the systems of Yoga and Vedanta.

Student: Once I have chosen a particular technique for meditation, how long should I work with it to determine if it is effective for me?

RH: If you practice seriously and regularly, once or twice daily, you will know within several weeks.

Another Student: You said that we cannot really judge whether or not we are making progress—and that we shouldn't try to judge. How do we know if the technique we've chosen is a good one for us?

RH: Any technique to which you are attracted and which

does not create a disturbance or conflict will be effective. As I have stated, most of the techniques are preliminary to learning to withdraw the mind and senses and achieve a degree of steady one-pointedness. The techniques of Hatha Yoga—asana and pranayama—are usually extremely helpful in this regard. When this one-pointedness has been accomplished, the "Who Am I?" or "Where Am I?" inquiry should be undertaken. The alternative to this inquiry is total self-surrender.

Student: Can I undertake the "Who Am I?" without any preliminaries?

RH: Of course. But if this should prove difficult and you cannot hold the mind steady and prevent it from flowing outward, do not abandon the inquiry. Work with the other techniques and continue to return to the inquiry.

Student: Is any preliminary practice required for self-surrender?

RH: No.

Student: Can you do both the surrender and the inquiry?

RH: One is sufficient. Put your energies into one. Later you will recognize that they are the same path.

Student: If you choose to "surrender," do you still meditate passively?

RH: You can. Sit quietly and surrender to the guru within.

Student: Do animals seek Self? What is their level of understanding? Do they evolve into human form and increase their understanding in this evolution?

RH: Did an animal come to you and ask you about Self?

Student (Smiling): No, but if you want to know the truth, my most constant companion is my dog. Perhaps I should instruct him in Yoga.
(Laughter)

RH: Leave your dog alone. Animals know who they are. Trees and flowers know who they are. Stones know. Only humans believe that they don't know who they are. Your dog can instruct you in "who you are" better than you can instruct him.

Student: Are you serious?

RH: Of course. Observe him closely and you will note spontaneous action without endless plotting and scheming in the hope of fulfilling illusory promises generated by an ordinary mind.

Student: From time to time I attend classes in sensory awareness, on awakening the senses and really getting in touch with those things in the world and in yourself that are usually not "sensed" in their fullness. Do you think this is beneficial?

RH: From our point of view, if these classes help you to understand the nature of the senses so that they may be more easily controlled and withdrawn as necessary, then they are beneficial. But if your objective is to sharpen the senses so that they may better perceive and increase your gratification in the world, then it is simply a case of your desiring to have a clearer image of illusion. In our work it is of no consequence whether one sees the illusion vaguely or sharply. *Determining the point of origin of the senses* is what must be done.

(There was an interval of silence.)

Students whom I have known for some years will come and tell me of their "progress." They will recount how they have overcome such-and-such bad habits, how their marriage or love life has improved, how they have achieved success in their various enterprises, and how they have had important insights into something regarding their practice which they formerly failed to understand. Frequently, I perceive that what has actually occurred is that certain concepts of ordinary mind have been supplanted by other concepts. The ordinary mind is in just as much control as it ever was; it has, in its resourcefulness, simply raised the game to the second power. The student is still deluded with progress." He sees himself moving forward toward a "goal," and because he has eliminated a bad habit, improved a situation, or had an insight into something, he is satisfied with his "progress." But he has only moved from one point on the circumference of the circle to another. He is just as far from the center at his new point on the circumference as he was at his previous one. All points on the circumference are equidistant from the center. I mention this here so that you will be aware of the ordinary mind's *illusion* of progress. "Progress," as it is understood in the world, has no application to meditation. One can truthfully say that he has "progressed" in his practice of the asanas and pranayama, but not in meditation. Either you are in the center, functioning as Self, or you remain on the circumference. You cannot make progress *toward* the center; you can only jump in completely, all at once. So remain aware that ordinary mind will frequently attempt to ingratiate itself by informing you of your "progress." But it has no intention of relinquishing its position of dominance, and while it is telling you of how you have eliminated a bad habit, it is sprouting a whole tree of new bad habits; while it is congratulating you on your insights, it is weaving a new web of entanglements to conceal from you the nature of maya. The crux of the matter is this: never be deceived by what ordinary mind is interpreting as "progress." Its "progress" is simply movement from one point on the circumference to another; in this way you are led to believe that things are "happening" and you are effectively kept off balance. Therefore, *be relentless in your pursuit of the source of that entity which is claiming the "progress."*

Another Student: I remember your stating in one of your books that the process of Self-recognition was more like a transformation, like a moth evolving into a butterfly.

RH: Yes. The beginning student who finds imagery helpful can think of his growth in Self-awareness as a metamorphosis, rather than in terms of stepwise progress. But this is merely an expedient for the novice. None of these limiting words and images can possibly depict the UNLIMITED.

Student: If, during meditation, a fly lands on your face, or you begin to itch, should you chase the fly away and scratch where it itches, or should you attempt to ignore these types of distractions?

RH: For your passive meditation practice it is best to select a place in which minimal distractions will be experienced. If you are absorbed in your meditation and a fly alights on your face, you will be oblivious to it. If you are not as yet completely absorbed, you will feel the fly, and it is natural for you to chase him away. How will it further your meditation if you are bothered by the fly but pretend that you're not? Nothing is gained in this work by ignoring discomfort or by any type of pretension.

Student: Is the same true of the legs when you're meditating in one of the Lotus positions?

RH: Of course. When you have reached the limit of comfort in the Lotus, remain for approximately one minute beyond this point. In this manner you will gradually increase the length of your sitting time.

Student: Isn't it peculiar how people who are serious about their spiritual development are often accused by their relatives or closest friends of being "unrealistic"? I have been told on a number of occasions that I'm turning my back on reality.

RH: Well, I think we've discussed this in sufficient depth for you to have the Yogic perspective of such matters. When the conspirators detect a threat, they will react accordingly. All who exist in maya, in the illusion, are *un*realistic. They have mistaken the unreal for the real and participate in a benign conspiracy to prevent this unreality from being exposed. Those who are awake to

Self do not know the self and its illusion, the world. All those who are awake to the world are asleep to Self.

Another Student: Suppose that one has intermittent experience of Self. When he is functioning in the world without the real sense of Self, but with just sort of a memory or impression of the experience, does he function in a way that is different from the way he did prior to his Self-experience?

RH: He *knows*—in a way that cannot be articulated—that he is not confined to a body and that he is not the doer. But the discharge of his duties proceeds as always. Why should this change? He is like an actor who gives the same performance each night at the theater. Although he knows that he is not, in "real" life, the character whom he portrays on the stage, this in no way affects his performance. And even if there should be a radical change in his "real" life, he adheres to the dictum "The show must go on." His performance on the stage is, therefore, unaffected. In the same way, your performance of your duties is unchanged. Usually, as the sense of "I am the doer" decreases, the world observes that your efficiency and the quality of your work increase.

Student: And what about when your sense of Self is absolute?

RH: Then you Know Absolutely that you are not the doer; you neither act nor reap the fruits of the action.

RH: I see that it's just about time for us to conclude our final discussion of this workshop. Permit me to make a few closing remarks.

First, listen to this quotation from the *Hatha Yoga Pradipika*: "As long as the mind does not assume the form of Self without any effort, so long is all the talk of knowledge and wisdom merely the nonsensical babbling of a fool." The point is that *practice* is the thing. All we have said and done here during this week is just so much smoke if it does not precipitate your serious, patient, and regular practice. Consider, once more, your situation in the mayic condition. [Mr. Hittleman read the following passage from his book *Yoga: The 8 Steps to Health and Peace*.]

"You find yourself existing in a dimension of constant threat and danger. You are beset on all sides by endless problems which, in your delusion, you attempt to resolve with the very instrument that creates them. You seek to Know and Understand, but you cannot because you are eternally separated, in a subject-object relationship, from that which you would Know. Through a universal conspiracy—in which you unknowingly participate—you accept these situations as 'the natural course of events,' as 'life.' Hypnotized by the self-appropriated authority of ordinary mind, immersed and believing in not only one but many 'selves' which ordinary mind manufactures and maintains, you subscribe unquestioningly to its illusory propositions. Among these fantasies, the doctrine of *desire-action-fulfillment* convinces you that it is natural and necessary to strive for happiness, success, pleasure, and security, that such elusive objectives can be achieved through the right kind of action, and that somehow your achievements can be made permanent. So, dutifully complying with the party line of the conspiracy, you experience incessant desires that compel you to undertake the incessant actions dictated for their gratification. But because your desires are interminable, because your actions can never truly satisfy these desires, and because you seek what is ultimate and permanent in a state where only constant impermanence and fluctuation obtain, you suffer. You suffer throughout not only this lifetime, but throughout an infinite number of lifetimes."

How does one awaken from this illusion, this dream of self, to that Reality which is his/her true and eternal nature? By total abandonment of all that is of the not-Self. *Self-recognition* has been the theme of this workshop and we have spoken in detail of the pertinent techniques. So, there is really nothing more to be said, is there? Go home and practice and let nothing deter you from practice.

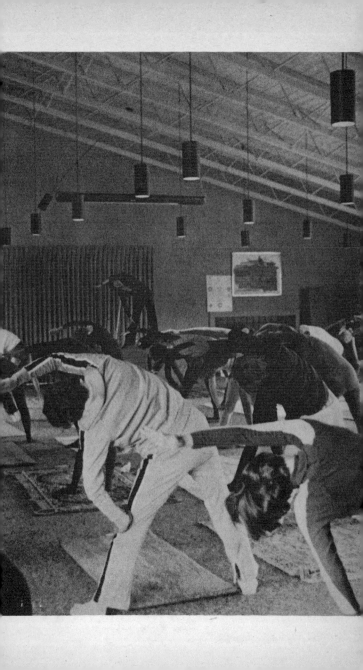

Permit me to close with this quotation from the *Siva Samhita*: "When this body which you now inhabit—which has been obtained through karma—is made the *means of obtaining Liberation*, only then does the carrying of its burden become fruitful; not otherwise."

Shanti! Peace!

Hatha Yoga

Students attending the workshop received intensive training in Hatha Yoga. Although classes were offered for the three categories of students—elementary, intermediate, advanced—the instructors of these classes emphasized the value of the *asanas* (postures) and *pranayama* (breath control) in the practice of meditation.

Mr. Hittleman has stated: "The body and the ordinary mind are one entity. They exert a direct and constant influence on each other. When the mind is disturbed, a corresponding dis-ease manifests in the body. The converse is equally true: a body that is ill-at-ease causes the mind to be even more agitated than it is in its usual restless condition. Because the *asanas* have an immediate quieting effect on not only the physical, but the subtle body, they can be of great assistance in helping the student to achieve that steady, one-pointed state which is essential for fruitful meditation." Consequently, it is certainly in the reader's interest to gain some proficiency in Hatha Yoga, regardless of which spiritual "path" he has chosen. Performing only those five techniques that are suggested in the Meditation Session section of this book can be of significant aid.

During several of the Hatha Yoga classes offered at the workshop, Mr. Hittleman assisted instructors in correcting students during their performance of various postures. I kept a record of these corrections and noted the errors that were most frequently made. The photographs in this section depict both a composite of errors and the correct position for each posture. The reader who is practicing Hatha Yoga at home should find these photographs particularly valuable because it is easy to overlook certain imperfections if she/he is not being continually observed by a qualified instructor.

Specifically, this Hatha Yoga instruction is offered:

1. To assist those who have not previously practiced Hatha Yoga, but who may now be inclined to determine what effect such practice has, particularly in regard to meditation. These readers may utilize only the five postures that are suggested in the Meditation Session section, or may undertake to experiment with all the techniques depicted. If these techniques are found to be effective, and the reader wishes to pursue the practice in greater depth, she/he should consult those books of Mr. Hittleman which present detailed instruction in the postures.*

2. To assist those practitioners of Hatha Yoga who wish to perfect their postures. These students should first perform the postures in their accustomed manner, and while in the final position of each posture, or immediately upon completion of the posture, study the photographs carefully to determine if they are committing one or more of the depicted errors. (The book may be placed in a position which will permit the student to see the photographs with minimal adjustment of the body while in the extreme pose of a posture.)

---

*Introduction to Yoga, Yoga 28 Day Exercise Plan and Yoga: The 8 Steps to Health and Peace.

⌐┐ CHEST EXPANSION
forward position

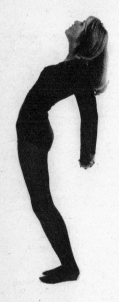

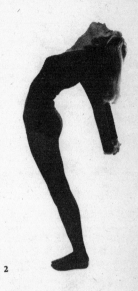

1

2

INCORRECT

Knees are bent.

Arms are not raised sufficiently high.

Head is not dropped back a sufficient distance.

Eyes are not looking directly upward.

CORRECT

Knees are straight.

Arms are raised as high as possible and remain in that position throughout movements.

Head is back as far as possible.

Eyes are looking straight upward.

1 CHEST EXPANSION
backward position

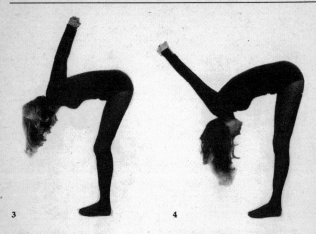

3

4

INCORRECT

Knees are bent.

Arms are not forward a sufficient distance.

Neck is not relaxed; head remains too high.

CORRECT

Knees are straight.

Arms are forward as far as possible.

Neck is relaxed; forehead is aimed at knees.

RISHI'S POSTURE

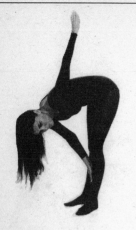

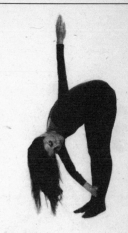

5

6

INCORRECT	**CORRECT**
Feet are too far apart.	Feet are close together.
Right leg, *not* left leg, should be grasped by right hand.	Hand holds inside of the corresponding leg; grasp is firm and as far down the leg as possible.
Leg should be held on *inside*, not on front; grasp should be very firm.	
Knee is bent.	Knees remain straight.
Upraised arm is too low and hand position is incorrect.	Upraised arm is straight upward, at an exact right angle with the floor.
Head is not turned a sufficient distance; eyes are not looking at upraised hand.	Head turns as far as possible to the left so that eyes may be fixed upon the back of the upraised hand.

Movements are performed on both the left and right sides.

3 TRIANGLE

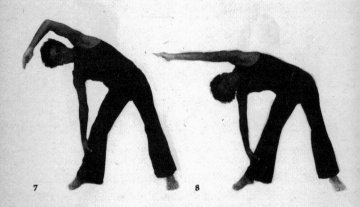

7   8

INCORRECT

Knees are bent.

Left arm is bent at elbow and is not parallel with the floor.

Neck is not relaxed; head is not lowered.

CORRECT

Knees remain straight.

Left arm is parallel with the floor.

Neck is relaxed; head is lowered as far as possible.

Right hand has firm grip on right calf; holding the calf firmly assists in lowering the trunk to the extreme position.

Movements are performed on both the left and right sides.

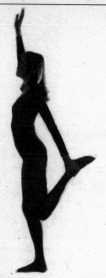

9

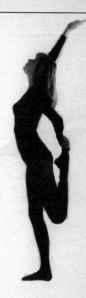

10

INCORRECT

Raised leg is too far away from trunk and is not raised sufficiently high.

Hand is holding foot at ankle rather than at top of foot.

Upraised arm is not back; fingers are apart.

Head is not back; eyes are looking frontward.

CORRECT

Hand holds top of foot (toes) and pulls leg up as far as possible, simultaneously holding it close to body.

Upraised arm moves backward as far as possible; fingers are together.

Head drops back and eyes look upward.

Movements are performed on both the left and right sides.

COMPLETE BREATH STANDING

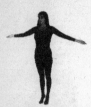

11

12

half-way position

Most students are able to perform these movements without significant errors. However, difficulty is frequently encountered *in coordinating the inhalation and exhalation with the body movements*.

The lungs should be completely emptied with a deep exhalation before beginning any movement. Following the exhalation, a deep inhalation is begun and, simultaneously, the arms are slowly raised.

At the half–way position of Figure 11, the lungs are half full and the body has risen partially on the toes.

completed posture

In the completed position of Figure 12, the lungs have been filled to capacity, the hands meet overhead (elbows straight), and the body is fully raised on the toes. The breath is then retained for a count of 10 to 20 seconds with the body held motionless.

The deep exhalation is then coordinated with the body movements so that the lungs are being emptied as the arms are slowly lowered to the sides (palms facing downward) and the soles of the feet are slowly lowered to the floor.

The lungs are fully emptied as the hands touch the thighs and the soles are fully on the floor.

Without pause the next inhalation is begun.

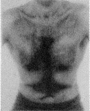

13

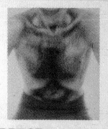

14

INCORRECT	**CORRECT**

The lungs have not been fully emptied; consequently, there can be only a partial lift of the abdomen. Figure 13 depicts what is more of a *contraction* than a *lift*. The contraction is not without value, but it does not provide the greater benefits of the full lift.

The lungs have been fully emptied so that the complete lift is possible. No air is permitted to enter the lungs while the lift is executed. Note the deep indentation in the jugular notch and compare it with the partial indentation of Figure 13. The deep indentation of Figure 14 occurs automatically when the lungs remain empty and the lift is performed.

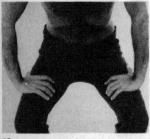

15

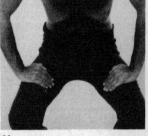

16

INCORRECT

Thumbs are hooked on sides of thighs; fingers are spread.

Palms are not pressed firmly against thighs.

CORRECT

All fingers are together.

Palms are pressed firmly against thighs with increased pressure during each lift.

ABDOMINAL LIFT

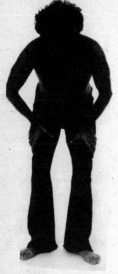

17

18

INCORRECT

Trunk and head are bent over rather than being held straight and simply lowered.

Knees are not sufficiently bent.

Hands are turned outward rather than inward.

CORRECT

Figure 18 depicts the Abdominal Lift performed correctly in all details.

The trunk is lowered and the knees bent as though the model is in the first stage of sitting down.

Remember that the abdomen is "snapped" out with a forceful muscular movement following each lift, rather than being allowed to simply relax.

7 TWIST
front view

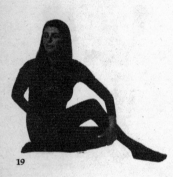

19

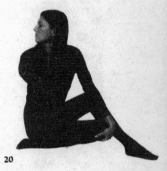

20

INCORRECT

Left hand has reached *around* the right knee rather than *over* it.

Head is not turned to the extreme right; consequently, the twist is incomplete.

Sole of the right foot is not fully on the floor.

Trunk is not erect.

CORRECT

Left hand holds left knee in a position that requires the left forearm to exert pressure on the right knee.

Head is fully turned to right.

Entire sole of right foot rests firmly on floor.

Trunk is held erect throughout movements.

7 TWIST
back view

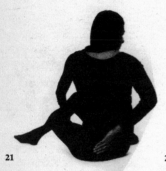

21

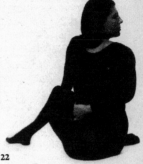

22

INCORRECT

Right hand is simply resting on the back rather than firmly holding the left side of the waist.

Note again the incorrect positions of the left arm, right foot, and head, and the curvature of the spine.

CORRECT

Right hand holds the left side of the waist.

Note again that the entire sole of the right foot rests on the floor; the head is turned to the extreme right; the trunk is held erect.

Movements are performed on both the left and right sides.

8 ALTERNATE LEG PULL

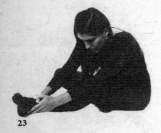

23

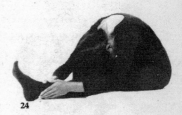

24

INCORRECT

Left knee is bent (which can be caused by the opposite foot being incorrectly placed; see Figure 25).

Spine is insufficiently curved.

Neck is not relaxed; head is not down.

Elbows are straight.

Hands are not gripping the ankle tightly to assist in downward pull of trunk.

CORRECT

Left knee is straight.

Spine is totally curved.

Forehead is aimed at knee or rests on knee; neck is relaxed.

Hands grip ankle (or foot) firmly and elbows bend outward; both these techniques assist in the lowering of the trunk.

Outstretched leg is always relaxed, never tensed.

Movements are performed on *both* the left and right sides.

⑧ ALTERNATE LEG PULL

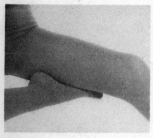

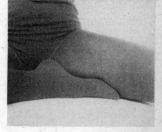

25

26

INCORRECT

Sole of foot is under thigh, rather than against it, causing knee to be raised.

Heel is away from perineum.

CORRECT

Heel is in the area of the perineum and the entire sole of the foot presses against the uppermost inside of the thigh.

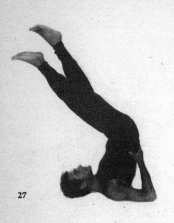

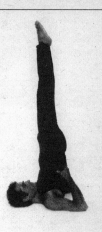

27   28

Although it is acceptable that the student not remain rigid and can relax the body during a Shoulder Stand, which is held beyond 3 minutes, Figure 27 depicts an undesirable degree of relaxation as well as a number of common errors.

It is always beneficial to have the chin either touching or as close to the top of the chest as possible.

The legs should remain together (although not necessarily rigid) unless the Shoulder Stand variations are being performed.

The trunk should not be permitted to slump into the angle depicted in Figure 27.

(The above instructions are for those who have achieved a degree of proficiency in the Shoulder Stand. For those who are beginners, any angle of inversion is acceptable.)

Figure 28 depicts the Shoulder Stand being performed correctly in all details. The point of concentration is on the breathing, which has been deliberately slowed, but which remains rhythmic and regular at approximately 2 to 3 breaths per minute.

10 PLOUGH

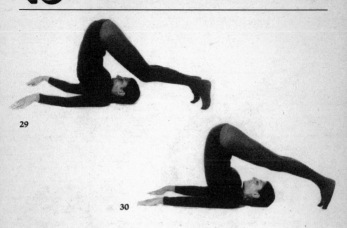

29

30

INCORRECT	CORRECT
Knees are bent.	Knees are straight.
Arms are too far apart; palms are raised from floor.	Arms are aligned with sides of body; palms are placed firmly against floor.
Legs and feet are apart.	Legs and feet are together.
Feet are placed too far behind the head, so there is insufficient curvature in the lumbar.	Feet are placed as close to the head as is possible while maintaining knees straight so that emphasis is felt in the lumbar.

11 BACK STRETCH

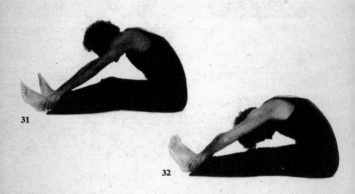

31

32

INCORRECT

Knees are bent.

Spine is insufficiently curved.

Elbows are *not* bent.

Neck is not relaxed; head remains too high.

Feet and legs are not together.

CORRECT

Knees are straight.

Spine is curved.

Elbows are bent outward as far as possible.

Neck is relaxed; head drops down as far as possible.

Feet and legs remain together; toes point upward.

12 SIDE RAISE

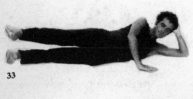

33

34

INCORRECT	CORRECT
Legs are apart.	Legs remain together throughout the lifting movements.
Legs are being raised in front of the trunk.	
Right hand is away from trunk; fingers are spread and pointing away from trunk.	Legs are aligned with trunk during lift.
	Right palm rests firmly on the floor close to the trunk and fingers point toward opposite arm.
Left palm is against back of head rather than supporting side of head.	Left palm supports head by being placed against left ear.

Movements are performed on both the left and right sides.

13 COBRA

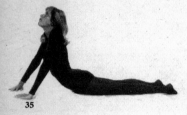

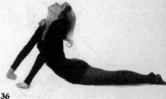

35   36

INCORRECT	**CORRECT**
Fingers are spread and pointing away from trunk.	Fingers are together and pointing directly toward the opposite hand.
Spine is insufficiently curved.	Extreme curvature of the spine.
Head is not in backward position.	Head is back as far as possible, with eyes looking upward.
Legs are held tensed.	Legs are relaxed throughout movements.
	Arms must be aligned with sides. If hands are placed too close together, the groin will leave the floor in the fully raised position; if the hands are too far apart, the trunk cannot be raised the distance that is necessary to effect the extreme curvature of the spine.

14 LOCUST

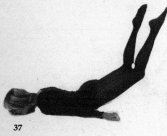
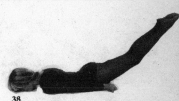

37   38

INCORRECT	**CORRECT**
Fists are placed so that all fingers are touching the floor.	Fists are placed on sides so that only thumbs and index fingers rest on floor.
Arms are too far away from legs.	Arms are adjacent to sides of trunk so that fists touch thighs prior to lifting of legs.
Knees are bent.	Legs remain together.
Legs are apart.	Knees bend only slightly.
Point of chin (rather than ball of chin) is resting on floor.	Ball of chin (and lips, if comfortable) rests on floor. If point of chin contacts floor, the height of the lift is decreased.
The lungs have not been half-filled prior to raising of legs.	The lungs have been half-filled prior to raising of the legs; air is retained during the interval of the lift and exhaled *after* legs have been lowered.

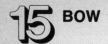

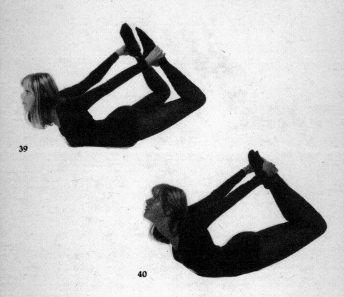

39

40

INCORRECT	**CORRECT**
Knees are apart.	Knees are together throughout movements.
Head is insufficiently raised; eyes are not looking upward.	Head is up as far as possible; eyes are looking upward.
Hands are holding feet too close to ankles.	Hands are holding tops of feet.
Trunk is insufficiently raised.	Trunk (and knees) is raised as high as possible.

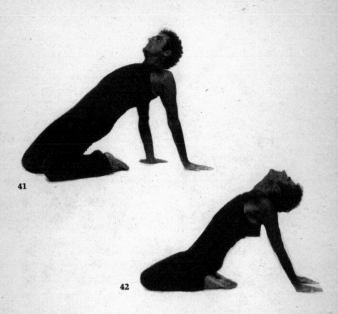

41

42

INCORRECT

Arms are too far apart, not aligned with sides; fingers are spread and pointing at incorrect angle.

Buttocks are not resting on heels.

Knees are apart.

Head is not in backward position.

CORRECT

Arms are aligned with sides; fingers are together and pointing directly away from trunk.

Buttocks remain on heels throughout movements.

Knees are together.

Head drops as far backward as possible; eyes look upward.

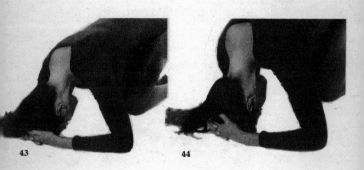

43 44

INCORRECT	CORRECT
The front area of the scalp rests on the floor and part of the head is actually *on* the hands.	The fingers are firmly interlaced and the sides of the hands rest rigidly on the floor.
The fingers are weakly interlaced and the hands are not being held rigidly.	The top and part of the back of the head are cradled against the hands.
	Forearms and elbows are also firmly placed on the floor.

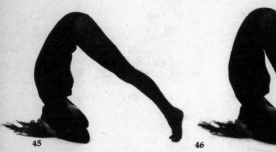

45

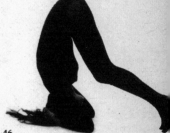

46

Both of the positions depicted in Figures 45 and 46 are correct. However, it is necessary to note here that the position of Figure 46 is often omitted by students and they attempt to move directly from Figure 45 into the position of Figure 47 (next page) without bringing the knees in close to the chest as shown in Figure 46. If the position of Figure 46 is omitted, the transition into Figure 47 cannot be effected smoothly; the student is forced to fling the legs unevenly upward, hoping to find the correct point of balance. This results in a hit-and-miss situation and is not in the Yogic spirit of smoothness and control. Consequently, the sequence of Figures 45, 46, and 47 must be performed.

17 HEAD STAND

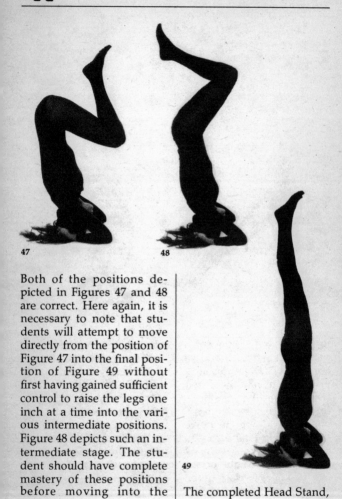

47

48

Both of the positions depicted in Figures 47 and 48 are correct. Here again, it is necessary to note that students will attempt to move directly from the position of Figure 47 into the final position of Figure 49 without first having gained sufficient control to raise the legs one inch at a time into the various intermediate positions. Figure 48 depicts such an intermediate stage. The student should have complete mastery of these positions before moving into the completed Head Stand.

49

The completed Head Stand, correct in all details.

18 SIMPLE POSTURE

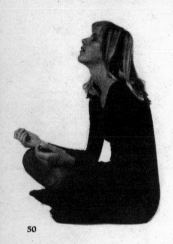

50

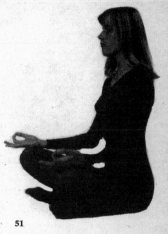

51

INCORRECT

The posture is without strength.

Trunk is not erect.

Head is held too high and is tilted; nose is not aligned with navel.

Fingers are bent; thumbs and index fingers are touching in the *mudra* without firmness.

CORRECT

Trunk is erect; abdomen is slightly distended.

Head is centered; nose is aligned with navel.

Eyes are *not* completely closed.

Thumbs and index fingers meet firmly; remaining fingers are together and forcefully extended.

The posture should emit strength and power, without tension.

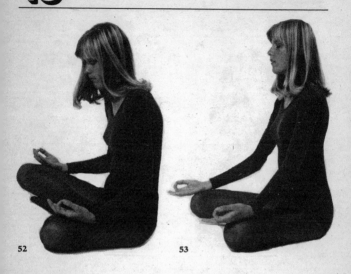

52   **53**

INCORRECT

Sole of right foot is not turned sufficiently upward and heel is not touching pubic bone.

Spine is curved.

Hands are on thighs rather than knees; finger position is weak.

Head is lowered and not centered.

Eyes are closed.

CORRECT

Sole of right foot is turned as far upward as possible.

Trunk is erect, abdomen is slightly distended.

Backs of hands are on knees; thumbs and index fingers meet firmly; remaining fingers are together and forcefully extended.

Head is centered; nose is aligned with navel.

Eyes remain partially open so that a slit of light may enter.

20 **FULL LOTUS**

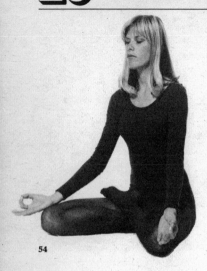

54

The Full Lotus, correctly performed. Left leg is on top and both heels are drawn in to touch the groin. Soles are turned upward as far as possible. Other details are identical with the Half-Lotus.

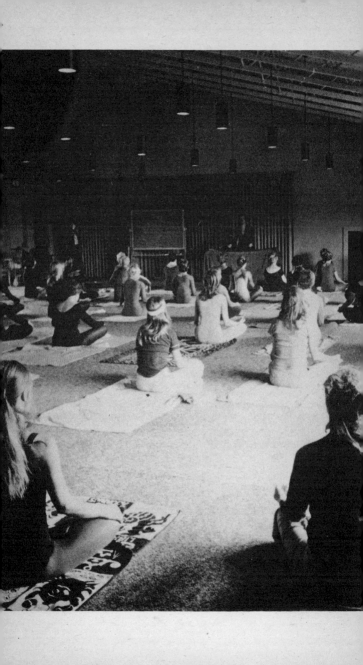

Meditation Practice

The following techniques comprised the basic early-morning meditation session at the workshop. The routine of asanas and meditation was designed for an interval of approximately 30 minutes.

1. Each of five postures was performed twice. The first execution was very moderate to gently stretch the body; the second was more advanced, but still not extreme because of the early hour. The usual holding periods in each posture were observed, but without breath retention or *yantra* visualization. (The visualization, breath retention, continuous-motion routines, etc., were included in the regular 90-minute mid-morning and mid-afternoon Hatha Yoga classes. These techniques may be learned from those books of Mr. Hittleman listed in the bibliography.)

The final position of each of the five postures is depicted in the following pages to refresh the memory of the reader who may wish to engage in meditation by following the routine of the workshop.

(1) Complete Breath　　**(2) Chest Expansion**

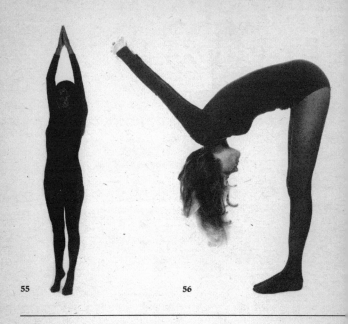

55　　　　　　　　　56

(3) Back Stretch

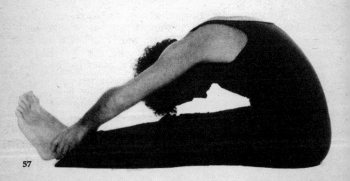

57

(4) Twist

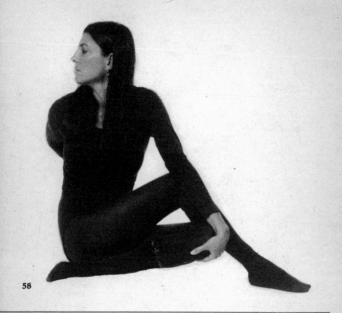

58

(5) Cobra

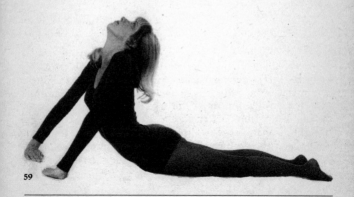

59

2. According to their ability, students then assumed one of the three cross-legged positions. Students were carefully checked by the instructor to make certain that the position of the entire body was correct in all details. (If students experienced discomfort of the legs during the meditation period, they were instructed to quietly stretch the legs straight outward, massage them at the knees for a few moments, and then return to the original position, *but with the legs reversed*. This was to be accomplished with as little disruption as possible.)

Simple Posture

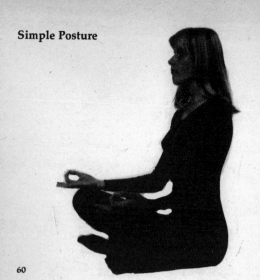

60

Half-Lotus

Full Lotus

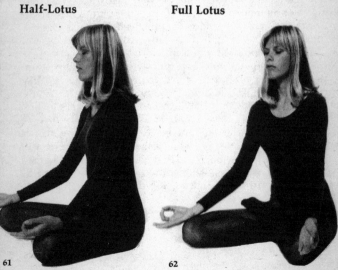

61

62

3. Next, approximately 2 minutes were spent in Observation of the Breath. Students were instructed to become aware of their breathing and to direct their undivided attention to it. The technique is practiced by excluding all thoughts and making the breathing pattern the sole focus of steady, one-pointed attention. (The practice cannot be timed by students, but they quickly get the feeling of approximately 2 minutes, or become aware of the fact that their attention is remaining steadily fixed upon the breathing. At this point they may proceed to the next meditation technique or, if they wish, continue with the breath observation. If the student elects to continue with the breathing technique, he relinquishes *observing* and traces the breathing to its source, to that place from where it arises and to where it goes. This is the technique suggested by Mr. Hittleman upon retiring for the night, just prior to sleep.)

4. Finally, the student undertakes the "Who Am I?" inquiry, or whatever he has chosen as the "seed" of his meditation: a yantra, OM, self-surrender, the listening for inner guidance, etc.

The passive-meditation interval was approximately 15 minutes in these workshop sessions. (Students practicing at home may spend as long an interval in passive meditation as they wish. Fatigue or discomfort—not restlessness—should indicate the termination of the practice period. The various dynamics of this were discussed by Mr. Hittleman during the meetings and appear in the text.)

Additional points mentioned by Mr. Hittleman, and directed to students who are practicing meditation at home, were: the selection of a location for practice where minimal distractions are likely to occur; the advantage of practicing at the same time each day; not to meditate for at least one hour after a meal; use of the same mat each day for practice.

He also reiterated, on several occasions, the importance of not looking for "results" or attempting to evaluate one's "progress." "Just practice seriously, regularly, and patiently," he stated. "All the value is in the *practice; the practice evolves into the goal.*"

Bibliography

Bhagavad-Gita. Any edition. (The definitive treatise on Karma Yoga.)

Blofeld, John. *The Zen Teaching of Huang Po*. Grove Press, New York, 1958. (A Zen Buddhist classic.)

Hittleman, Richard. *Guide To Yoga Meditation*. Bantam Books, New York, 1969.

———. *Introduction To Yoga*, Bantam Books, New York, 1969. (Instruction in elementary and intermediate Hatha Yoga.)

———. *Yoga: The 8 Steps To Health And Peace*. Deerfield Communications, New York, 1975; Bantam Books, New York, 1976. (The philosophy and techniques of the six major Yogas; includes *yantra* visualization.)

Nityaswarupananda, Swami. *Astavakra Samhita*. Vedanta Press, Hollywood, California, 1969. (A superb summary of Advaita Vedanta, the philosophy of nonduality.)

Osborne, Arthur. *Ramana Maharshi and the Path of Self-Knowledge*. Samuel Weiser, New York, 1970. (Mr. Hittleman regards Ramana Maharshi as the foremost teacher of this century.)

Patanjali. *Yoga Sutras* (or *Yoga Aphorisms*). Any edition. (The primary reference work for the student of Yoga.)

Hatha Yoga Pradipika
Siva Samhita
Gheranda Samhita

The editions suggested by Mr. Hittleman of the above three classical Hatha Yoga texts are Allahabad, 1914 and 1915, reprinted in 1974 by AMS Press, 56 East 13th Street, New York, N.Y. 10003. It is usually necessary to order these books through a bookstore. They are excellent translations from the Sanskrit, but expensive; the prices should be checked before ordering.

The Yoga For Health television series can be seen in many areas of the country. Readers who are interested in receiving a listing of Mr. Hittleman's various publications and instructional recordings may write to:

Yoga For Health
P.O. Box 475
Carmel, CA. 93921

Bantam Book Catalog

Here's your up-to-the-minute listing of every book currently available from Bantam.

This easy-to-use catalog is divided into categories and contains over 1400 titles by your favorite authors.

So don't delay—take advantage of this special opportunity to increase your reading pleasure.

Just send us your name and address and 25¢ (to help defray postage and handling costs).